Warfare in World History

The immediate effects of war can be catastrophic, but wars have also proved to be the most important instruments of long-term change in world history. This text is the first of its kind to survey how warfare has developed from ancient times to the present day and the role it has played in shaping the world we know.

Warfare in World History covers the major periods of military history, each delineated by new advances in technology and the unique social, political and cultural contexts in which its wars were fought. The periods discussed include:

- the pre-gunpowder era;
- the development of gunpowder weapons and their rapid adoption in Western Europe;
- the French Revolution and the industrialization of warfare;
- the First and Second World Wars;
- the Cold War and the wars of liberation fought across the Third World.

With in-depth examples illustrating the dominant themes in the history of warfare, *Warfare in World History* focuses not only on the famous and heroic, but also discusses the experiences of countless millions of unknowns who have fought in wars over time.

Michael S. Neiberg is Associate Professor of History at the United States Air Force Academy. He is the author of *Making Citizen-Soldiers* (2000).

Themes in World History
Series editor: Peter N. Stearns

The *Themes in World History* series offers focused treatment of a range of human experiences and institutions in the world history context. The purpose is to provide serious, if brief, discussions of important topics as additions to textbook coverage and document collections. The treatments will allow students to probe particular facets of the human story in greater depth than textbook coverage allows, and to gain a fuller sense of historians' analytical methods and debates in the process. Each topic is handled over time – allowing discussions of changes and continuities. Each topic is assessed in terms of a range of different societies and religions – allowing comparisons of relevant similarities and differences. Each book in the series helps readers deal with world history in action, evaluating global contexts as they work through some of the key components of human society and human life.

Gender in World History
Peter N. Stearns

Consumerism in World History:
The Global Transformation of Desire
Peter N. Stearns

Warfare in World History
Michael S. Neiberg

Warfare in World History

Michael S. Neiberg

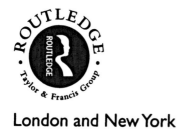

London and New York

First published 2001
by Routledge
2 Park Square, Milton Park, Abingdon, Oxon, OX14 4RN

Simultaneously published in the USA and Canada
by Routledge
270 Madison Ave, New York NY 10016

Routledge is an imprint of the Taylor & Francis Group

Transferred to Digital Printing 2005

Typeset in Garamond 3 and Gill by
Keystroke, Jacaranda Lodge, Wolverhampton

British Library Cataloguing in Publication Data
A catalogue record for this book is available from the British Library

Library of Congress Cataloging in Publication Data
Neiberg, Michael.
    Warfare in world history / Michael S. Neiberg.
        p. cm. – (Themes in world history)
    Includes bibliographical references and index.
    1. Military art and science—History. 2. Military history. I. Title. II. Series.
U27 .N45 2001
355′.009—dc21   2001019950

ISBN 0–415–22954–5 (hbk)
ISBN 0–415–22955–3 (pbk)

Contents

Acknowledgments   vii

Prelude: 5 June 1944   1

1   The classical age (to 500 CE)   9

2   The post-classical period (500 to 1450)   21

3   The emergence of gunpowder weapons, 1450 to 1776   34

4   Nationalism and industrialism   46

5   World War I   59

6   World War II   73

7   The Cold War and beyond   85

    Conclusions   99

    Index   103

Acknowledgments

I am grateful to the series editor, Peter Stearns, for suggesting that I write this book and for his comments on various versions. My friend and colleague Dennis Showalter was kind enough to read the entire book and his thoughts made this book a much better product. John Jennings and Jim Tucci shared their vast knowledge of East Asia and the ancient world, respectively, with me. Michelle Moyd helped me with finer points of African history. Thanks are also due to Mark Wells, Jeanne Heidler, Vance Skarstedt, Paul Bauman, Ben Jones, Mark Erickson, Bill Astore, and Paul Merzlak who took time to sit down and discuss military history with me. If any errors remain, they are mine alone.

I also want to thank my wife Barbara for her endless patience at battlefields, libraries, and museums around the world. I dedicate this book to our daughter, Claire, in the hopes that warfare will, for her generation, be always a remote and arcane subject best left to history books.

Prelude: 5 June 1944

American General Dwight Eisenhower sat in his headquarters near Newbury, England and considered the poor weather outside. The Western Allies – Americans, Britons, Canadians, Poles, Belgians, Italians, Czechs, and Free French – had placed a force of 200,000 men, 6,000 ships, 13,000 vehicles, and 5,000 fighter aircraft under his command. One hundred and sixty-three air bases had been specially constructed to maintain supporting air operations. This immense force was scheduled to depart for the invasion of the Normandy region of northern France in just a few hours. For months, Allied pilots had bombed railways, roads, and bridges to isolate Normandy from German reinforcements. Airborne units had been trained to land at key points by parachute and by glider. General George Patton, whom the Germans feared more than any other commander, had been put in charge of a fictitious First US Army Group, complete with false radio traffic and foam rubber barracks, to deceive the Germans into thinking that the landing would come further east. British engineers had created two "mulberries," artificial harbors (each the size of the English port at Dover) that used six miles of steel roadways, each capable of unloading more than 7,000 tons of supplies per day.

All of that effort was put at risk by the twenty knot winds, six foot waves, and cloudy skies of a summer storm in the English Channel. The bad weather Eisenhower saw outside his window was his worst nightmare. To go now under such dismal conditions could put the entire operation, codenamed "Overlord," in grave danger. Eisenhower knew that the operation was risky enough under ideal circumstances. The Germans, under Field Marshal Erwin Rommel, had prepared a formidable series of defenses known as the Atlantic Wall to repulse any Allied attempt to land in northern France. More than 4,000,000 mines, hundreds of machine guns, thousands of miles of barbed wire, and scores of concrete pillboxes awaited the Allies across the Channel. Any additional risk could kill thousands of Allied soldiers and possibly destroy the Allies' best chance to liberate occupied France.

But not going posed great risks as well. Russian leader Joseph Stalin had been begging and pleading for a "second front" in France for two years. The Russians had already lost untold millions of soldiers and civilians bearing the brunt of Germany's war machine. The Allies had assured Stalin, after repeated delays throughout 1943, that he would get his second front in spring, 1944. If Eisenhower ordered a halt now, the Allies would not be able to go again for at least two more weeks, when tides and moon phases would again be optimal. Soldiers were already confined to marshalling areas, pilots to their hangars, and sailors to their ships. If the attack were delayed two more weeks, could the Allies continue to keep the gigantic operation a secret?

All of these factors weighed on Eisenhower's mind; the decision was his alone. His generals and admirals gave him conflicting advice. After meeting with his chief meteorologist, Eisenhower turned to his advisors and calmly said, "OK. Let's go." Southern England turned into a flurry of activity. Planes roared to life, ships disembarked, and soldiers heard Eisenhower's message: "The eyes of the world are upon you. The hopes and prayers of liberty-loving people everywhere march with you." BBC radio broadcast the second line of the French poem "Chanson d'Automne," the signal to the French Resistance that the hour had arrived to start destroying bridges and cutting telephone lines that could be useful to the Germans. The Allies were coming.

D-Day is, for good reason, one of the best known events in military history. One extraordinary man's decision and thousands of ordinary men's heroism changed the course of European, American, and world history. D-Day combines all of the critical elements of military success: resources (human and material) appropriate for the task at hand; an organizational scheme that makes maximum use of those resources; leadership to direct those resources; and coordination of forces, each making its own distinct contributions. Almost 40,000 Allied soldiers died liberating Normandy, but they created a second front that, along with renewed Russian offensives, ended World War II in Europe within a year.

The elements that decided events in Normandy have their parallels on thousands of battlefields across space and time. Technologies change, leaders change, and war itself changes, but the essential role of warfare in world history has remained an important constant. Wars alter basic patterns of societies over both long and short runs and concentrate dynamic change within very short periods of time. This book will examine warfare and its many changes from the dawn of history to the present day. It is not my intention to glorify or celebrate war, but to explain how it has changed and why it is important as an actor and a force for change in world history.

War can be defined by three essential dimensions: violence; legitimacy; and legality. All wars are violent. All are based on the premise that force is necessary to achieve a desired aim. It has become commonplace in contemporary society to speak of a "war on poverty" or a football game as a "sixty minute war." These constructions, of course, miss the point entirely. Warfare necessarily involves the mass application of *lethal* force. Armies, navies, and air forces are trained to deliver maximum lethality as efficiently as possible. To do so, they must overcome moral and ethical standards that abhor killing. That in turn means that men and women raised to believe that killing is wrong must be provided with sufficient motivation to ignore those teachings.

War's legitimacy helps to convince soldiers, sailors, and airmen that killing in certain contexts is not only not wrong, but may, in fact, be rewarded. War is unlike criminal violence or mob activity because it derives legitimacy from a political, societal, or religious source. Men are, in effect, given license to ignore commonly accepted societal conventions against killing and destroying. Most organized religions reserve special afterlife rewards for those men who die in a sanctioned war. Christian Crusades and Muslim Jihads are perhaps the best known examples, but ancient Meso-American, South Asian, and Celtic religions also offered warriors immortality and/or a rewarding afterlife.

Odd though it may seem, wars involve legality. All wars, even so-called "total" wars, are fought within understood sets of rules. In Medieval Europe, special courts enforced these rules, specifying, for example, that the knight who seized his enemy's right gauntlet was his rightful captor and thus deserving of whatever ransom he could negotiate. The contemporary practice of shaking right hands upon meeting someone emerged from this gesture between "men of honor." The Geneva Conventions and Hague Treaties that govern war today are a product of these rules. Often, these codes and laws remained unwritten, though as in European chivalry, Chinese *li* or Japanese *bushido*, they could be extremely elaborate. War is not, then, a free-for-all of killing. It is carefully governed and regulated by both armed forces and the societies they serve.

A history of warfare therefore involves looking at much more than armies, navies, and air forces. It also involves looking at economic, social, political, and cultural patterns in civilian societies as well. War is one of humankind's most complex institutions and it must be so understood if it is to be understood at all. This book can only give a brief introduction to war and introduce some of the many key issues in the history of warfare.

The chapters that follow in this book are divided into seven periods: the classical period, which includes the Greeks and Romans; the post-classical period; the age of gunpowder weapons; the age of industry; World War I; World War II; and the Cold War period. Trying to fit the entire history of human conflict into these seven chapters necessarily forces grouping disparate events together. Nevertheless, historians must periodize in order to make sense of the past. The wars of each of the periods listed above share enough commonalties to allow us to consider them together. Indeed, shifting patterns of warfare help chart and explain some of the big changes in world history more generally.

We will further divide each chapter into three sub-chapters: the men; the weapons; and the battles. I will use the phrase "the men" because the overwhelming majority of combatants in the history of warfare have been male. I ask the reader to forgive my gender-specific terminology. It is important to keep in mind, however, that male domination of the battlefield does not mean that women have played no important roles in warfare. As we will see, by World War II women had become absolutely indispensable to the successful prosecution of warfare.

Our study of "the men" will involve an examination of who they were, why they fought, and how they organized themselves. Recently, historians of warfare have understood "the men" to mean much more than the senior commanders. Recent research has led to a vastly increased understanding of the "common" soldiers and the way that armies have organized them to fight. Their recruitment, training, and treatment have had substantial impacts on the way that armies and navies have fought. To focus exclusively on generals, admirals, and heads of state correspondingly overlooks critically important factors.

Systems for organizing men into fighting units have changed tremendously over time. In modern societies, sharp distinctions separate "military" and "civilian" spheres, but this organization is neither natural nor automatic. Thirteenth-century Mongols, noted one historian, belonged to a society in which "there was no such thing as a civilian." For every type of society humankind has developed there is a corresponding type of military. They share in common the need to meet military challenges while at the same time staying true to their society's dominant cultural, political, and social beliefs. One of the key reasons to consider war as a world history theme is that it both reflects and causes some of the key features of the civilizations that define so much of the world historical panorama.

No single system of military recruitment exists, but several general types have dominated. Three of the most common are: the citizen-soldier (motivated by allegiance to their country or region); the professional (motivated by money); and the conscript (motivated by fear). As their name implies, citizen-soldiers are men with a political, economic, and social stake in the society they serve. Often they are organized into locally-based militias. They are rarely full-time soldiers. Ordinarily they have little time to devote to formal training but, in theory, their close connections to their societies give them a moral and emotional edge over their enemies, especially if they are fighting to defend their own society. Militias are inexpensive because they only need to be assembled in times of crisis, but, for that very reason, they rarely possess a vast wealth of military expertise.

Professional soldiers spend most of their lives learning the military art. They are ordinarily highly skilled and often equipped with advanced weapons. They can be citizens of the society they serve, but do not need to be. Mercenaries, men who serve only for money and who are generally not otherwise connected to the society they serve, have been a common solution to military procurement problems throughout time. Because they must be paid a salary (and often a pension) and equipped, professional soldiers of all kinds are expensive to maintain. When they do not receive promised payments, moreover, they can become disloyal. This problem is especially prominent with mercenaries.

The final method for getting men to serve in the military is to compel them. Coercion can take many forms, from impressment and slavery to mandatory national service laws. In some cases, though by no means all, men will cooperate with coercive military systems out of a sense of civic obligation. If men see themselves as playing a role in national goals that they share (as most men did in World War II) they are unlikely to resist the system, even if it is coercive. Such a system can have much in common with the first system, but in this case the men are not "pure" volunteers. Some threat of punishment exists to compel them.

If they do not see linkages between their enforced military service and national policy goals, draft resistance and outright refusal to comply may follow. A conscript army of this type is often less expensive than a professional one because if men are serving primarily out of fear of punishment there is no need to spend lavishly to keep them happy. Conscripts are therefore not always as highly motivated as men procured through voluntary systems. If they are truly serving against their will, conscripts might very well see the institution conscripting them as their real enemy.

These systems can co-exist in a single society or blend together according to the culture and politics of a given society. Men can, of course, serve for a combination of financial and patriotic reasons. The important point here is that the system of personnel procurement matters for determining the performance and character of an army or navy. No single system is necessarily "better" than another. Each has its own strengths and weaknesses.

A history of warfare also involves a careful look at commanders. Wars force leaders, both civilian and military, to make quick decisions that mean life or death for thousands. The right person, appearing at the right time, and making the right decision, can change history. One of his rivals reportedly once said that Napoleon's personal appearance on a battlefield counted for 30,000 men. Wars create extraordinary circumstances wherein the decisions of one person can alter a society forever. The fate of western Europe hung in the balance of Dwight Eisenhower's simple "OK. Let's go" command.

Similarly, an analysis of "weapons" involves looking at military resources of all kinds. Some historians argue that superior weapons and other technologies (transportation and communication technologies like landing craft and radar, for example) alone are enough to guarantee victory. General Eisenhower certainly had at his disposal a tremendous pool of resources from the simple child's "cricket" click toy (used by paratroopers to find each other after their drops) to sophisticated B-17 bombers. Resources can mean a new, decisive weapons technology like the atomic bomb or a technology as seemingly simple as an accurate map.

Technological and production advantages certainly help the side that possesses them, but resources rarely determine the outcomes of wars by themselves. As we will see, more technologically sophisticated societies do not always defeat less sophisticated ones. Militaries must be able to introduce new technologies into their doctrines and employ them on the battlefield in an effective manner. Doing so involves careful applications of civilian economic resources and making intelligent choices about what kinds of technologies to develop.

Finally, we will examine how all of these elements came together on the battlefield. It is there that empires have been made and lost; heroes born and killed; and history fundamentally changed, in some cases in just a few short hours. It is there that men, organization, and technology meet their ultimate test. As we will see, the battlefield has always been chaotic, lethal, confusing, and disorienting. But the soldiers who marched with Genghis Khan in the thirteenth century would not have recognized the industrial battlefields of World War I. We must understand how what one historian called "the face of battle" has changed if we are to understand warfare.

As the previous discussion should make clear, war is an infinitely complex activity. It touches the basic economic, cultural, political, and social beliefs of society. It is serious business, often practiced over the centuries by men and women who have dedicated their lives to it. This book will introduce you to war and the ways it has changed from the era before gunpowder to the age of atomic weapons, but it can only be an introduction.

One last set of definitions will help. Wars, campaigns, and battles are often analyzed along three dimensions: strategy, operations, and tactics. Put (too) simply, strategy is the where and when; operations are the who; and tactics are the how. To take our D-Day example once again, strategy involved choosing to attack Normandy on 6 June 1944 as opposed to, say, Norway or Belgium in July. Operations divided the attack zone in Normandy into five separate beaches, two American, two British, and one Canadian, each with its own supporting naval task force and air arm. Tactics dictated a prelanding naval and air bombardment at each beach followed by an amphibious assault by a division or two of infantry. Keeping these definitions in mind will help conceptualize large military operations and understand how they evolved.

War's origins

Exactly where, when, and how man first went to war remains a mystery. Recent research by archeologists and anthropologists suggests that virtually all societies in all parts of the world have engaged in war. Totally peaceful societies have been the clear exception. Enlightenment philosopher Thomas Hobbes (1588–1679) argued that war was a result of man's individual need to protect himself from the many enemies he faced. Men entered into formal and informal protection agreements with their neighbors in order to provide for their mutual defense. These agreements eventually led to the creation of states and armies. Organizing and planning with others led to greater security, though it could also lead to more organized violence.

Other philosophers, such as Jean-Jacques Rousseau (1712–1778), argued that man, in his original state, was peaceful. He "learned" to fight wars as his societies grew more sophisticated and more hierarchic. Man, in Rousseau's view, is not naturally violent. Violence is a consequence of the process of societal development. For Hobbes, the reverse was true. Man, naturally violent, created organizations to ameliorate or prevent chaos.

Recent research supports Hobbes's view of the origins of war more than it does Rousseau's. Archeological and anthropological evidence demonstrates that warfare predates civilization. Man in his natural state was rarely, if ever, peaceful. Neolithic civilizations produced elaborate fortifications and have left evidence of corpses obviously killed in organized battle and often buried in mass graves. In other words, even before men and women learned how to write, farm, or construct permanent shelters, they learned how to organize themselves to fight their enemies.

Precivilized warfare could be highly intense and terribly violent. Many precivilized societies mobilized a greater proportion of their young men to fight than many civilized societies would do later. The Maori people (who live in modern-day New Zealand) mobilized approximately twenty-eight per cent of their men for war against each other and later against Great Britain. During World War II, by contrast, the Soviet Union mobilized twenty-two per cent and the United States mobilized seventeen per cent. Precivilized weapons like slings and bows evolved from hunting weapons and were often much more deadly in the hands of skilled practitioners than western small arms until the development of rifled muskets in the nineteenth century.

One anthropologist has concluded that prehistoric people most often fought wars for religious reasons or to avenge an insult from another society. Wars of this nature were usually short, as societies could not go to war at every perceived insult. The unwritten rules of precivilized warfare dictated that a single revenge killing in battle could avenge the insult and thus end the war. In this sense, early warfare might be violent, but the direct death rates were usually low. Wars also occurred for control of arable land, especially as a given region's population growth outpaced its supply of good land or access to some precious commodity like fresh water. Contemporary wars for control of scarce oil resources have parallels in precivilized wars for control of water, salt, or good grazing grounds.

The development of more organized warfare depended on a variety of factors including competition for scarce resources, the existence of an agricultural surplus (which in turn freed up some men to focus on soldiering), and societal growth. As societies grew, they developed more sophisticated record keeping systems and authority structures. These systems allowed for the management of larger and larger groups of soldiers. On the battlefield, these systems of organization often translated into greater operational and tactical complexity as well.

Nevertheless, several factors limited war: terrain; religion; weather; supply; and wealth. In some societies, like the Aztec, the purpose of war was to take prisoners to be ritually sacrificed to the gods by whose grace the Aztecs believed they had inherited the Toltec legacy. Religious and political restrictions forbade the killing of a man on the battlefield unless absolutely necessary. Aztec weapons were therefore designed to wound rather than kill. Warfare thus fit into a given society's dominant belief systems.

The Aztec example illustrates the important point that societies could, and did, limit the destructive powers of their own military systems. Still, as political systems grew more sophisticated, so did military systems. Civilization (defined as urbanization, the development of writing systems, and a division of labor) could provide a society a tremendous military advantage. In fact, civilization and military sophistication often developed together. As political elites commanded a monopoly or near-monopoly over their society's military power, their political power naturally grew as well. Similarly, as political power grew, so did the resources and organizations necessary to build and maintain military forces. As states grew, so did armies. As armies grew, war became more important.

We can, therefore, assume that man in his precivilized or prehistoric state understood and experienced war. In the "classical period" which we will examine next, societies developed elaborate religions, bureaucracies, languages, political structures, and social systems. They also developed increasingly sophisticated military systems. The age of Julius Caesar, Alexander the Great, and the Great Wall of China left military legacies that continue to influence warfare to this day.

Chapter 1

The classical age (to 500 CE)

Thermopylae, 480 BCE

Traditional rivalries between the Greek city-states and the Persian Empire flared into war in the fifth century BCE. The Greek city-states themselves often fought one another, but in this case they united to resist the commonly despised Persians. A combined Greek army under Athenian leadership stopped the Persian's first attempt to invade Greece at the Battle of Marathon in 490 BCE. Through spectacular leadership, the Athenians inflicted 6,400 casualties on the Persians at a cost of less than 200 Athenian dead.

Ten years later Persian King Xerxes set out to avenge his father's loss at Marathon and punish the Greeks for their resistance. Persia was then the largest empire in the world, with armies many times larger than any combination of Greek city-states could field. Xerxes sent an army of overwhelming numerical superiority into Greece hoping to end the conflicts once and for all and extend Persian influence into southeastern Europe.

To stop Xerxes' 200,000 man army, the Greeks needed time to call their militiamen into service. Greece had only a small 7,000 man force of Spartans and their allies under the command of General Leonidas to slow the Persians down and buy needed time. To improve his chances of success, Xerxes sent his best troops, the Immortals, to smash this first line of Greeks. Leonidas needed to find a place where, in the words of one historian, "Greek lives could be sold most dearly." Knowing that he and his men would not return, he chose to bring only men with children, thus ensuring that at least family names would survive.

Leonidas chose to defend a mountain pass near Thermopylae so narrow that only one cart could go through at a time. In places, the pass was less than 15 feet wide. Leonidas led his men to the far side of the pass, then feigned a retreat to entice the Persians inside. Once in the pass, the Persians could not use their superiority of numbers. Fighting in shifts, 300 Spartans and 700 allied soldiers held the Persians at bay in the pass for two days until a farmer told Xerxes of another mountain pass. Now surrounded, the Greeks were slaughtered. The Persians decapitated Leonidas and placed his head on a pole as a trophy of their success.

Only one Spartan survived the battle, but the heroism of Leonidas and his men bought the Greeks enough time to organize naval forces and win the Battle of Salamis later that year. Having lost more than 200 ships to the Greeks' forty, the Persian armies were isolated and cut off from resupply. Greek armies also dealt the Persians a land defeat at Platea the following year, forcing the Persians to call off their campaign. Leonidas' stand made Greek victory possible. Rather than being lauded as a hero, however, the lone survivor of that battle was shunned as a coward and later committed suicide. The Spartans expected their soldiers to win battles or die trying.

Thermopylae demonstrates the predominance of disciplined infantry on the classical world's battlefields. Although each civilization handled military affairs in its own distinct fashion, all relied on foot soldiers trained to act in unison. As the classical empires grew, they came increasingly to rely on these infantry forces to protect what they had conquered and to extend their influence even further. The growth of the classical civilizations necessarily occurred simultaneously with the growth of warfare.

The men

The classical period saw important evolutions in the development of states and civilizations. With these developments came concurrent evolutions in the nature and roles of armies. These armies developed differently in Europe and in Asia. Political and philosophical differences between the great classical civilizations led to differing approaches to the problems of fighting wars. All of the classical civilizations relied on infantry as the main means of fighting, but significant similarities generally end there. For this chapter, we will focus on how traditions of warfare and military force, many of which still influence us today, developed in Greece, Rome, China, and, to a lesser extent, India.

The expansion of civilization permitted much more sophisticated forms of organization, specialization, and economic support. Ancient Greece was among the first civilizations to turn these developments into military advantages, though as we will see it was not the only one to do so. By the eighth century BCE, warfare was an integral part of Greek society. From the poorest yeoman farmer to the most prestigious elites, military service literally defined the course of a man's life and his importance to his society. The famous Athenian tragedy writer Aeschylus asked that his epitaph mention not his plays, but his service at the Battle of Marathon.

Greek city-states, in constant competition with one another and constantly threatened by the Persians, built significant military power. Sparta kept a body of coerced laborers called helots to perform manual labor and farming. As a result, Spartan citizens could devote their time exclusively to military service, itself necessary to keep the helots from rebelling. All male Spartans owed military service to their polis and all women bore the responsibility of producing future warriors. At age seven Spartan boys left their parents' home and began military school. Weapons training began at age twelve. By age twenty the men were ready to enter a military unit called a mess. Members of a mess ate, trained, and slept together forming close bonds that paid dividends in combat. At age thirty a man became a full "equal" in his mess.

Sparta's obsessive devotion to military training was the exception. Most Greek soldiers (like their peers around the world) were farmers who assembled when an enemy force threatened their territory. Because most Greeks were not professional soldiers, their military system had to be simple. In battle, Greek soldiers formed dense groupings called phalanxes that were usually eight to sixteen men deep. Phalanxes, when packed together, provided an impressive wall of heavily armed men. For the phalanx to succeed, the men had to practice rigid discipline; if the phalanx broke, all of the hoplites might well be killed. Greek military systems thus depended on close links between the men who fought. These links normally preceded military service itself, as most of the men came from the same region and therefore knew each other well. Military leaders led from the front of a phalanx and often died in battle.

The man who finally beat the Greek system was a Macedonian and one of the greatest military minds of all time. Alexander the Great sought to eliminate, not just defeat, his enemies. After leading a successful, though grueling, six-month siege of the city of Tyre, Alexander killed 8,000 Tyrians and sold the remaining 30,000 into slavery. He always led his armies personally, directing charges that time and again nearly led to his own death. His use of flexible, fast arms like cavalry and light infantry wreaked havoc on the slow Greek phalanxes. Over the course of eight years, he defeated every enemy in his path and created an empire that spanned 3,000 miles before his men, homesick and out of worthy foes, begged him to return to Macedonia. Alexander's success is partly a function of his using infantry in combination with slings, archers, and light cavalry.

The Roman system intentionally copied many Greek and Macedonian features, including rigorous discipline and training. As novices, Roman soldiers trained with wicker and wood replicas of weapons that were twice as heavy as real weapons. They built up physical fitness with long all-weather runs and marches that continued throughout a career that lasted as long as twenty-five years. They also trained in skills like camp construction, learning to use a small shovel called a *dolavella* with which Roman soldiers built defensive works. While on campaign, Romans typically dug in every night. A virtual army of support personnel followed, including veterinarians, blacksmiths, and doctors.

The ideal Roman soldier developed the same close links to his comrades that the Greeks had possessed. Until the second century BCE, only landowners could serve in the Roman legions, thus replicating the Greek system of putting the men with the most at stake in the army. The concept of citizens (though not necessarily landowners) dominating the army survived much longer, though Rome did employ non-citizens in certain areas like archery. Many of these men could attain Roman citizenship upon successful completion of military service.

Despite all the similarities to Greek warfare, the Romans differed from the Greeks in their understanding of leadership. Greek leaders understood themselves to be "first among equals," usually equipped and treated just like their men. By contrast, Roman generals in the empire period became so powerful that their men often swore oaths of loyalty to them personally. Generals like Julius Caesar turned their armies into virtual empires of their own. This system provided generals with the operational flexibility they needed in an empire as large as Rome's, which counted 60,000,000 by 1 AD. When the generals fought amongst themselves, however, the system could, and did, devolve into civil warfare.

Chinese generals rarely held the power and independence of western generals. Asian understandings of warfare shared the western focus on disciplined infantry, but included a more highly developed bureaucratic state control over military affairs as well as a more intense study of strategy and military philosophy. The fifth century BCE writer Sun Tzu wrote what many believe to be the first important work on strategy and theory, *The Art of War*. His principles are still studied today the world over. Sun Tzu outlined many military doctrines that remain familiar to any soldier including surprise, mobility, flexibility, and deception. *The Art of War*, later revived by Mao Tse Tung in China, formed the basis of many guerrilla doctrines in the twentieth century.

After the Spring and Autumn Period (722 BCE to 481 BCE), ancient Chinese armies were normally much larger than those in Greece. As early as the third century BCE one Chinese army contained almost one million men. In a 295 BCE battle, 240,000 men died. Most of these men were peasants who had been transformed into infantrymen. The Chinese, like the Greeks, instilled intense discipline and wrote the first drill manuals. The Chinese delayed introducing cavalry until the third century CE in part because horsemanship required the rider to abandon noble robes in favor of "barbarian" short trousers and shirts.

The Qin Dynasty (256 to 206 BCE) resembled the Roman Empire in many of its military attributes. It used military power to consolidate and extend its imperial power, thus laying the groundwork for the Han Dynasty, one of the important classical civilizations. Between 232 and 221 BCE the Qin Dynasty conquered an area that stretched from modern-day Vietnam to the famous Great Wall, itself a Qin project. Military efficiency was critical to Qin expansion. In 1974, a farmer near the city of Xi'an (the Qin capital) found the tomb of the first Qin emperor. It contained 8,000 life-sized terra cotta warriors and horses that guarded the tomb. The warriors are a symbol both of the power of the Qin and the importance of the military to the dynasty.

Unlike the Romans or the Greeks, however, the Chinese believed that violence was only one part of warfare, and not necessarily the most important or most useful. Sun Tzu and others argued that the purpose of military power was to induce your enemy's compliance, preferably peacefully, by using whatever means were available. Surprise, deterrence, deception, and intelligence were among viable options to fighting a pitched battle. The powerful

Han Dynasty (206 BCE to 220 CE) discredited "wu," the art of warfare, in favor of "wen," the art of peace. The Han introduced competitive exams and fitness reports, written by civilians, as requirements for promotion. Civilians managed supply and determined military assignments.

Also unlike the Romans or the Greeks, Confucian Han China believed that the moral absolute always rested on the side of peace. War, they believed, was unnecessary if the ruler did his job properly. As the Thermopylae case shows, western warfare adopted an approach that emphasized quick, intense battle. Whereas for the Greeks warfare was a central event in civic life, for the Chinese it was often an admission that all other resorts to solving problems had failed.

These early experiences led the Chinese to adopt three positions that would have been unfamiliar to the Greeks or the Romans. First, the Chinese tended to prefer non-violent means to resolving disputes. Warfare to the Chinese was not legitimate until all other possibilities had been rejected. An emperor's military success was, therefore, a shameful symbol of his moral and political weakness, not a proud statement of his martial prowess. Such a viewpoint would have been inconceivable to the Greeks and Romans who prized success on the battlefield above all else. Second, the Chinese preferred defense to offense, thus the Great Wall and the general weakness of Chinese naval forces. The Chinese often chose to wall off or pacify border nomads rather than fight them. Third, the Chinese were the first major civilization to subordinate the military to a civilian bureaucracy. Chinese emperors rarely had to fear that their generals were planning action against them.

India, too, developed important military traditions in this period, especially under the rule of Samudra Gupta (ruled 330–375) and his son Chandra Gupta (ruled 375–415). Samudra Gupta, called by one historian "the Napoleon of Ancient India," defeated nine kings in northern India and eleven in southern India to create a large empire with no south Asian rival. Chandra Gupta once assembled an army of 600,000 infantry, 30,000 cavalry and 9,000 elephants. He also set up a naval affairs office and one of the world's first secret services to gather intelligence about his enemies. India also produced the *Arthasatra* (*The Manual of Politics*), a guide to warfare that rivals Sun Tzu's *Art of War*. It advised Indian princes on the value of discipline and the importance of placing qualified men into leadership positions.

Military historians sometimes refer to the classical period as the age of infantry. All of the systems described above focused on infantry, though their motivations for creating such systems differed somewhat. Breeding of horses and the development of technologies like stirrups had not advanced far enough to allow cavalry to dominate, though the Chinese made extensive use of chariots in the Spring and Autumn Period. Infantry therefore dominated the age. Along with infantry-based military systems came many of the conventions that we still associate with the military, most notably discipline (to ensure that men did their jobs out of fear of punishment) and small-group solidarity (to ensure that they did not let down their friends and comrades). These conventions remain in practice today. Although the weaponry has changed, a classical army in its broadest outlines still has much in common with twenty-first century counterparts.

The weapons

All classical civilizations relied on weapons, such as javelins and slings, that evolved from weapons used for hunting as well as weapons, such as swords, specifically designed for warfare. As weapons evolved, so too did armor in response to men's desires to protect themselves. As we have already noted, superior weapons did not produce automatic victory on the battlefield, but they provided a tremendous advantage especially in the hands of well-motivated and well-trained men.

Greek hoplites provided their own equipment and weapons. Each soldier used a hoplon (the shield that gave him his name) that protected himself and his neighbor's right side inside a phalanx. Shields weighed as much as sixteen pounds, were made from as many as seven layers of animal hides, and were strong enough to stop a spear. The shield was shaped so that it provided no protection if the soldier put it on his back to cover him during a retreat. It worked only if a man charged forward with it. His bronze armor, breast plate and shin guards (called greaves) provided comprehensive protection from head to toe. It also weighed as much as seventy pounds (at a time when most Greek men weighed less than 150 pounds), limited vision, severely restricted movement, and could be quite hot. If men so armored were able to hold their phalanx together, however, they could form a virtually impenetrable barrier.

For offensive weapons, the Greeks relied on a six to eight foot long spear. Some armies, notably Alexander the Great's Macedonians, used a twenty foot long spear called a *sarissa*. The longer the spear, the more points that preceded the first line of men. Typically the first three to five ranks (depending on the length of spear used) would march with their spears pointing forward to create the stabbing power of the phalanx. Those in the back rows tilted their spears up at an angle to deflect enemy javelins or arrows. The only other weapon that the hoplite might carry was a short sword that was only good in close quarters if the phalanx broke apart.

The Greeks disdained enemies like the Persians and the Macedonians who preferred to fight from a distance. Lacking the discipline or superb bronze armor of the Greeks, the Persians used missile weapons like slings, javelins, bows, and crossbows to try to break the phalanxes apart. Alexander's Macedonians used the phalanx as well, but in a combined arms approach that also included cavalry, missile weapons, and light infantry.

This combination of short-range weapons and long-range (or missile) weapons existed in the east as well. The standard Chinese weapons, as in Greece, were the spear, and an axe called a *ko*. By the fourth century BCE the Chinese had developed crossbows with an effective range of eighty yards. One source claimed that in 209 BCE a Chinese emperor had 50,000 crossbowmen in his service. Even adjusting for the inaccuracy of many ancient sources, such an array of crossbowmen speaks volumes about the sophistication of Chinese weapons and the mass production required to make them. Around the same time, the Chinese also developed a primitive poison gas made from dried mustard. The Chinese, too, wore armor and carried shields, though they were more likely to be made of leather than the bronze preferred by the Greeks.

Many classical civilizations, most notably the Greeks, also developed navies, designed to deny the enemy his ability to resupply his land forces. A Greek warship, called a trireme, could have as many as 170 rowers in three layers. With top speeds approaching ten knots and a large bronze battering ram, a trireme could cut an opposing warship in half. At its height, Athens, Greece's supreme sea power, had a force of 40,000 rowers and more than 200 triremes. But fleets lacked navigational aids and fresh water storage; therefore they generally stayed within sight of land.

Unlike the Greeks, the Romans generally disliked naval warfare, despite their commanding geographic position on the Mediterranean Sea. Roman sea tactics usually came down to boarding enemy vessels and using standard land tactics on board ships. Instead of the sophisticated naval tactics of the Greeks, the Romans developed a series of planks and hooks to get their soldiers from their ships to those of the enemy. These tactics defeated Rome's chief naval rival, Carthage, in the First Punic War.

On land, however, the Romans excelled. They used a combination of weapons in a system that took maximum effect of all of them. Typically, Roman combat formations began with throwing spears called a *pila*. These ingenious spears had a center made of soft iron or light wood. Upon impact the soft iron center bent, making it impossible for the enemy to throw it back. After the battle, however, Roman smiths could reshape the weapons; thus the Romans had devised an early example of metal recycling. Ideally, attacks by *pila* would break up enemy formations, allowing the elite of the Roman army to advance with a short sword called a *gladius* with which to swing at exposed limbs. This system of combined arms proved to be remarkably effective in combat.

Like the Chinese, the Romans benefited from the tremendous engineering abilities of their civilization. Roman armies built roads to improve mobility, communications, and supply. As a result Roman legions could often depend on garrisons and supply depots to keep them fighting at an optimal level. Even today many of the major highways of Europe are reconstructions and improvements on the Roman system. The next important innovation in military land transportation technology would not come until the introduction of the railroad in the nineteenth century. The Romans also built walls and even diverted the course of rivers to improve operational effectiveness. Rome also excelled at several ancillary technologies such as medicine, construction (they invented concrete), and communications. The Romans divided their alphabet into five groups of five letters. Then, using two torches they developed a system for communicating across distances. The position of the first torch indicated which of the five groups contained the letter; the second torch determined the letter. The Romans also developed simple but effective codebooks to keep the enemy from divining the message.

Chinese engineering rivaled that of the Romans. The Qin Empire began a process of connecting existing walls to form a 2,000 mile-long barrier (known today as the Great Wall) to prevent nomadic incursions. Athens built a 200-yard wide double wall system to guard its links to the sea. The Romans also built walls, including Hadrian's Wall designed to keep Scots out of England. Field fortifications also developed, allowing soldiers to defend their camps and supply lines.

To defeat powerful fortifications, the ancients also developed complex siege engines such as ballistas and catapults capable of hurling stones and other objects (including dead horses to pollute water supplies) inside city walls. Demetrius of Rhodes used a device called a *helepolis* ("city taker") nine stories and 140 feet tall. It used 5,200 square feet of timber and had iron plates to protect it from attack as well as two interior staircases. It required more than 3,000 men to move it, but it allowed Alexander's troops to get close enough to jump off and get inside defended walls. It also protected them from the arrows, rocks, hot oil and hot sand that those inside poured onto the besiegers. Similar siege engines existed in other armies as well.

The Chinese (and to a lesser extent the Indians as well) used chariots. Each Chinese chariot had two horses, a driver (usually a noble), an archer, and a warrior armed with a *ko*. Chariots provided speed, but without infantry support they were extremely vulnerable. As a result, each Chinese chariot operated with as many as twenty-five supporting infantrymen. Gupta chariots in India were larger, requiring four horses and carrying as many as six men. Despite their speed, chariots proved to be unwieldy and difficult to maintain on campaign. As a result they steadily declined in importance over the classical period.

Animals constituted one more "technology" used by the armies of the classical period. Mounted warriors remained secondary to infantry, but when used effectively cavalry could add speed, shock, and pursuit. Animals also provided logistical support. One Indian army under Chandra Gupta used 9,000 elephants and 30,000 horses to support 600,000 infantry. Animals came with certain drawbacks, however, sanitation being among the most important. Forty thousand animals produce a lot of fertilizer. They also required a lot of fodder to feed them. In combat, moreover, elephants tended to scare easily and in their panic might kill men near them, regardless of which side they were on.

If this era represents the age of infantry, then the weaponry must be understood as the tools of the foot soldier. Spears, swords, shields, and axes dominated warfare. In response, armies developed heavy armor to protect their men as much as possible. Missile weapons like javelins and bows tended to be less central. The ancient foot soldier relied instead on bronze and iron arms and armor, making combat a furious contest of metal against metal and flesh.

The battles

Warfare formed an integral part of the creation of empires in this period – from Alexander the Great to Rome to Gupta India to Qin and Han China. Those civilizations that could convert their economic, bureaucratic, technological and political advantages into military advantages expanded at the expense of their neighbors. Those that could not often faced elimination at the hands of more powerful foes. Although many non-military factors explain the rise of the great empires in the classical period, it is a mistake to ignore the role that battlefield supremacy also played.

Greek warfare's organization came from the dominant economic and political patterns of the city-state system. Because their agricultural system was so sophisticated and productive, Greek city-states became aggressively territorial, both in protecting what they had and in coveting what others had. Intensive agriculture also produced large surpluses and a general sense of equality among the citizenry. Generals, like most other office holders in their society, were normally elected officials.

Because most of the weapons of this age required armies to get close to one another, classical warfare necessarily involved clashes of men at close quarter. The battlefield therefore became a loud, confusing, and quite fearsome place. Greek hoplite battles were simple, stark pushing and shoving matches. Because of the weight of Greek armor, men could not move easily nor could they see what was going on around them. Once a battle began, the noise of clashing metal made giving orders difficult. Thus many battles were decided by a short but violent clash between phalanxes. The weakest men took positions in the middle of the phalanx to be, in the words of Greek strategist Xenophon, led by the men in front and pushed by the men in back.

Few non-western societies shared the Greek fondness for quick pitched battles. Historian Victor Davis Hanson notes that the Greeks were willing to kill *and* die. To most non-Greeks (including the Persians) such an approach seemed foolhardy at best. The Persians were willing to kill, but were much less fond of dying. As a result, they tried to fight from further away with missile weapons to try to break up the phalanx. They also counted on longer operational campaigns to wear the Greeks out. As we saw from Thermopylae, the Persians had to engage the Greeks eventually, but they preferred to do so after their enemy had been worn down as much as possible.

After centuries of success, the Greek hoplite met his demise in 338 BCE at the Battle of Chaeronea at the hands of a young Alexander the Great, then serving as a lieutenant to his father Philip II. Philip and Alexander entered battle with 32,000 men to the Greeks' 50,000, including members of an elite Theban unit known as the Sacred Band. Philip's phalanx charged the Athenians on the Greek left flank, then, on cue, backpedaled. The Athenians counterattacked, leaving a hole in the center of their line. Alexander led a cavalry charge through the opening between the Athenians and the Thebans while another

Macedonian cavalry unit swarmed around the Theban right side, thus encircling the Sacred Band. When the Athenians looked back they saw that their Theban allies were surrounded. They panicked (the English word "panic" comes from the Greek attribution of fear to the deity Pan), breaking their phalanx and leaving them open to the vigorous attacks of the Macedonians. In one day, the Greeks lost 20,000 men. Macedonian combined arms destroyed the cumbersome Greek phalanx and left Philip and Alexander masters of Greece.

If the key to Greek (and to a lesser extent, Macedonian) warfare lay in the rigid and orderly phalanx, then the key to Roman warfare lay in a kind of disciplined and organized chaos. A Roman military unit looked to disintegrate its enemy by attacking with successive rows of differently-armed and differently-trained troops. As many as five separate waves of Roman soldiers using five different weapons systems might face the enemy. The Romans, through dedication and intensive training (to properly use a gladius required eight to ten months of difficult training), presented a constantly changing face of fresh troops alternatively armed with javelins, swords, and spears.

Few opposing armies could match the Roman system at its height. In particular, Roman tactical flexibility decimated Greek and Macedonian-style phalanxes, especially if the Romans could entice their opponents to fight on uneven ground as they did at Pydna in 168 BC. Still, the Romans were not invincible. Their most complete defeat came at Cannae in southern Italy in 216 BC, 122 years to the day after Chaeroneia. Few ancient battles have been so exhaustively studied for lessons in how to destroy, not just defeat, one's opponents with a single stroke. The great Carthaginian general Hannibal chose to fight the Romans in a narrow plain with a river to his left and a series of hills to his right. Geography limited the Romans' ability to maneuver and take full advantage of all of their arms, as it did to the Persians at Thermopylae. Hannibal placed combined units of infantry and cavalry on either flank and in the center placed a combined force in an upside-down U shape with the center bowed out toward the Romans. Hannibal hoped that the Romans would see the exposed center and try a frontal attack.

Hannibal guessed correctly. When the Romans charged, he put his plan into action. The center bent back, forming a cul-de-sac into which the Romans advanced. Then the two cavalry flanks moved in and trapped the Romans inside. For the rest of the afternoon, Romans died at the rate of 100 per minute in a killing cauldron that appalled even combat-hardened men. More than 50,000 Romans died that day. Cannae became a classic case-study in total victory.

Roman soldiers fought for patriotism and the greater glory of Rome. Indian warriors fought in part to fulfill their dharma, or caste obligations. The famous Indian text the *Bhagavad Gita* (or *Song of the Lord*, begun in the second century BCE) describes an epic war between two branches of a northern Indian family. One of the principle characters, Arjuna the warrior, is reluctant to kill members of his family, even though they are fighting on the other side. In the end, the deity Vishnu, disguised as Arjuna's chariot driver, convinces him that he must fight to fulfill the obligations of his caste. For a Hindu warrior in this period, fighting represented the fulfillment of God's will. Consequently, warfare, especially in northern India, tended to be formal and adhered to elaborate rules in accordance with its religious importance. As Gupta India grew more powerful, battle became less ritualistic and armies became larger.

The same general pattern holds in China as well. Warfare in the Spring and Autumn Period was mostly confined to the nobility. The ethics of the battlefield followed the code of propriety known as the *li*. Because the Chinese of this period understood war to be a contest between gentlemen, war was a ritualistic affair, with the *li* guiding the behavior of the combatants in a similar way to how chivalry would later guide battles in western Europe and *bushido* would guide battles in Japan (see Chapter 2). Infantry served primarily to support the noble charioteers and therefore armies remained relatively small, about 10,000 men at their largest.

The wars of the Spring and Autumn Period became increasingly destructive, necessitating changes in the nature of Chinese warfare. During the Warring States Period (403 BCE to 221 BCE) seven powerful states created mass armies; even the smallest of these states conscripted enough peasants to form armies of 100,000 men or larger. Cheaper iron weapons replaced the bronze weapons preferred by the nobility. The *li* no longer guided the actions of warriors, who were now overwhelmingly of peasant background.

By the end of this period, mounted warriors began to increase in strength. Better horse breeding on the steppes of central Asia led to powerful nomadic armies based upon cavalry instead of infantry. Although few realized it at the time, the Battle of Adrianople in 378 CE represented an important shift in military history. The Visigoths, a once impoverished people who sought charity from Rome, used cavalry to defeat an army of mostly Roman infantry. The barbarian victory at Adrianople should not be overstated; it did not, as some historians claim, destroy the Roman Empire. It did, however, underscore that by the fourth century the mounted rider had begun to replace the foot soldier as the dominant instrument of warfare. The great age of infantry was over.

Legacies

As they did in so many other areas, the classical civilizations left important legacies for the future of warfare. Across the globe, militaries grew increasingly more sophisticated, and established fundamental links with the cultural, social, economic, and political systems within which they operated. Warfare became absolutely integral to the development of governments and to civilization itself.

All of the classical systems relied on infantry and therefore needed to develop systems to control large numbers of men. Discipline became the method for forming effective military units out of bands of men. Even today, discipline remains the hallmark of military institutions worldwide. Messes and other systems also created a sense of small-unit dynamics. The classical armies seem to have figured out what later observers took to be a fundamental principle of military service: that men might be motivated by patriotism, religion, or the greater glory of their empires, but they fight primarily for the comrades in their small unit.

A careful reading of Sun Tzu, the *Arthasatra*, and the great Roman and Greek thinkers reveals that the basic principles of warfare and military strategy were carefully thought out thousands of years ago. Any serious student of the military is well served to start with these works. General George Marshall, who commanded American army forces in World War II, told a contemporary that one could not understand warfare without reading the Athenian general Thucydides, considered by many to be the first true historian. Thucydides traveled across Greece and spoke to Athenians and non-Athenians alike to write a complete, and, to the best of his abilities, impartial history of the Peloponnesian Wars. His writings, and those of Xenophon, who tried to finish the work Thucydides left undone upon his death, reveal the high level of strategic thinking among the ancient Greeks.

By 500 CE warfare had become one of the most important of all human activities. Armies and navies had the power and the ability to command considerable resources from the societies they served. Success or failure on the battlefield meant the difference between glory and annihilation. Warfare had become a highly organized and, in many cases, bureaucratic, operation, increasingly performed by professionals anxious to find ways to improve their trade and defeat their enemies. By the fourth and fifth centuries CE, the barbarians at the gate had solved the problem of defeating the Gupta, Han, and western Roman empires. As the collapse of these classical civilizations visibly demonstrated, no political entity could pretend to great power status without serious study of, and dedication to, excellence in warfare.

Further reading

Start with the classics, including Thucydides, *The Peloponnesian Wars* (New York, Modern Library, 1982); Sun Tzu, *The Art of War* (New York: Barnes and Noble, 1994); Richard Sawyer, ed., *The Seven Military Classics of Ancient China* (Boulder: Westview Press, 1993); Homer, *The Odyssey* (New York: Penguin, 1996); Homer, *The Iliad* (New York: Penguin, 1990); and Julius Caesar, *Caesar in Gaul and Britain* (Cambridge: Cambridge University Press, 1958). Excellent secondary works include Lawrence Keeley, *War Before Civilization* (Oxford: Oxford University Press, 1996); Victor Davis Hanson, *The Western Way of War: Infantry Battle in Classical Greece* (New York: Knopf, 1989); John Warry, *Warfare in the Classical World* (London: Salamander Books, 1998); Pierre Ducrey, *Warfare in Ancient Greece* (New York: Schocken Books, 1986); Graham Webster, *The Roman Imperial Army* (New York: Barnes and Noble Books, 1985) and Frank Kierman and John Fairbank, eds, *Chinese Ways in Warfare* (Cambridge: Harvard University Press, 1974).

Chapter 2

The post-classical period (500 to 1450)

Manzikert, 1071

In 1049, the Seljuk Turks, recent converts to Islam, invaded Armenia to challenge the power of the Christian Byzantine Empire, the eastern remnant of the Roman Empire. Beginning in 1067 a series of Seljuk raids devastated the Anatolian hinterland. Under the command of Sultan Alp Arslan (whose name means "Victorious Lion") the Turks then moved west and captured the fortified city of Manzikert, on the eastern edge of modern-day Turkey. Seeing his power threatened and fearful of a rising tide of Muslim dynamism, the Byzantine emperor Romanus set out to recapture Manzikert and force the Seljuk Turks out of Asia Minor.

Romanus' army encountered problems even before it arrived on the field of battle. His army of 60,000 men included soldiers from various, sometimes mutually antagonistic, communities. His Germanic troops at first refused to accompany him on the campaign. The Seljuk Turks, on the other hand, were more united as a result of their shared faith in Islam. Despite their smaller numbers (about 50,000) they were more energetic and better motivated than the polyglot Byzantines.

The Byzantine army looked little different in broad outline from the Roman and Greek armies of centuries before. Its strength was heavy infantry protected by an unreliable light screen of mercenary cavalry commanded by Romanus' main rival for Byzantine power, Caesar John Ducas. The Turks, in contrast, built their army around highly mobile light cavalry archers. Unlike the Byzantines, the Turks were quick and capable of delivering a missile attack quickly, and with great accuracy.

Once at Manzikert, the Turks originally fell back in the face of the Byzantine infantry, though this action may have been a ruse. Then, at dusk, the Turkish cavalry charged hard and fast at the flanks of Romanus' army, bending his line into a backwards "C." The Byzantine army's inferior cavalry deserted at the sight of the Turkish horsemen, leaving the slow heavy infantry with no protection. The Turks turned the Byzantine flanks, then attacked the unguarded rear. When it was over, every Byzantine soldier was either dead or prisoner. Romanus himself was brought to Alp Arslan and forced to agree to tribute payments for the next fifty years. His problems, however, were not yet over. Once released, he found that the deserter Lucas had taken power in Byzantium.

Manzikert made the Seljuk Turks masters of Anatolia and secured their northern flank for a drive on to the Holy Land. Their superior unity, based in Islam, and their tactical superiority, based on light cavalry, won the day. Turkish armies continued to move west, seizing more and more Byzantine territory. Finally, in 1092, the Byzantine emperor saw no choice but to plead for help. Three years later, with a call of "God Wills It," Pope Urban II launched the First Crusade. Thousands of Christian knights and common soldiers headed east with the twin goals of rescuing the Holy Land from Muslims and looting that same Holy Land to enrich their own purses. Manzikert set in motion a train of events that changed the political and religious maps of Europe and Asia forever.

Manzikert also demonstrates two important changes of this period. First, it proves that across Eurasia, most successful armies shifted their focus from infantry to cavalry as their main arm. Such cavalry units took several forms, from heavy, armored cavalry popular in western Europe to very light, but fast, cavalry among the Mongols. Militaries, like the Byzantine, that held to the classical pattern of infantry formations, suffered. Second, religion came to play a greater role in warfare, especially in the region from western Europe to India. This second theme is entirely consistent with the general spread of world religions in the post-classical period.

The men

In Europe and the United States, the post-classical period (defined here as the period between the collapse of the classical civilizations and the advent of effective gunpowder weapons) is frequently epitomized by the Arthurian knight. The image of the noble, Christian hero who adhered to ideas of loyalty and chivalry, continues to grab the imagination of popular culture and history alike. Nevertheless, it is mostly a myth. Only three parts of this image roughly reflect the reality of post-classical warfare: the dominance of cavalry over infantry; the role of religion in motivating warriors; and the reciprocal system of loyalty known as feudalism.

First, the mass usage of iron stirrups and horseshoes transferred centrality on the battlefield from the infantryman of the previous period to the mounted warrior. Stirrups allowed mounted warriors to shoot arrows or to deliver a blow from a lance with the full combined power of man and horse. Across most of Eurasia, cavalry took on an importance that it did not have in the ancient period.

A war horse and the accouterments that went along with mounted warfare were quite expensive; to equip and train a single knight required the revenue of 300 to 450 acres of land every year. Therefore, military power became concentrated in the hands of a select few. A mounted warrior needed at least three horses (because of the high loss rates on campaign and in battle), armor for himself and the horse, weapons, saddles, fodder, and squires to handle the horses. He also needed time to learn the complicated and intricate tactics and rituals of mounted warfare.

Warfare in this period was often characterized by plunder and looting, both as a way of intimidating one's enemies and as a way of making war profitable. Most often an army plundered its enemies, but in 1207 during the Fourth Crusade, the Byzantines' own allies could not resist the lure of the empire's wealth and sacked their capital city. Capturing one's enemy could also be a profitable enterprise. Knights frequently held other knights as prisoners of war until ransoms could be arranged. As noted in the introduction, a prisoner "belonged" to his captor if he removed the vanquished man's right gauntlet; from this gesture emerged the practice of shaking right hands. The Magna Carta, written in 1215, which limited the powers of the English king (who sat at the top of the feudal structure), nevertheless specifically permitted him to tax his vassals for the purpose of ransoming a knight once. Should he be unfortunate enough to become a prisoner twice in his life, it was up to his friends and family, if they could afford the ransom, to pay for his release. Elaborate tournaments also offered one the chance to make money. Victorious knights normally received the loser's armor, weapons, and horse as prizes.

Not all mounted warriors were knights. The Mongols, who created an empire from the Caspian Sea to the Pacific Ocean, based their military system on light cavalry. Using armor made primarily of silk and leather, their warriors could strike quickly and eliminate their enemies. Mongol boys often rode ponies before they learned to walk and lived within a system of total discipline. They used stirrups to enable them to fire arrows accurately while riding. They also used powerful composite bows and a device called a thumb lock to increase the bow's range to 350 yards.

Unlike most societies of the post-classical period, Mongol society was nearly completely militarized. They organized their hunts like military operations, with entire units engaged in surrounding prey. Early Mongol experience with horses paid dividends later. As adults, Mongols could often ride fifty miles a day or more when on campaign, providing unmatchable operational speed. Mongol skill at riding also allowed for the creation of a horse-based communications system, not unlike America's Pony Express of the nineteenth century. Alone among the societies under study here, Mongol women sometimes accompanied their men into battle, as the mother of the great Mongol leader Genghis Khan is believed to have done in campaigns against the Persians.

Light cavalry also worked well in the Middle East, where superior horses made the region an early convert to mounted warfare. Islamic armies used camels for operational mobility, permitting them to move as fast as twenty miles per day with little water. In combat, they often turned to high-quality Arabian horses.

Infantry never went away. The Christian armies of the First Crusade (1095 to 1099) involved 1,300 knights supported by almost 30,000 foot soldiers. But cavalry dominated; as the First Crusaders quickly learned, no foot soldier by himself could stand up to a fully armed warrior on horseback. Furthermore, foot soldiers lacked the knight's social status. Mounted warriors (most often nobles) disdained "common" foot soldiers. Archers, too, normally fell below mounted warriors on the social scale. For the knight, fighting commoners brought neither honor nor wealth, as infantrymen and archers could not be ransomed. Despite the social divides, post-classical mounted warriors needed infantry and archer support to succeed. On rare occasions, disciplined infantry was able to repel or even defeat cavalry. The exalted position of the mounted warrior, then, was a function of both military and social factors. This status reflected the general growth of decentralized aristocratic political systems in the post-classical period.

Second, except in East Asia, faith came generally to play a greater role in warfare, reflecting the growth of world religions in this period. The spread of Islam, in particular, inspired and broadened religious motivations for warfare. From Afghanistan to Spain and south into Africa, the success of Muslim armies led to a resurgence of military activity. The Crusades are perhaps the best-known manifestation of the role of religion in warfare, but many others exist as well.

By the ninth century, Islam, Christianity and Hinduism had inspired faith-based justifications of warfare. The Crusades represented a series of Holy Wars for opposing religious forces. The Christian crusades to the Middle East are best known, but crusaders went to Spain, Lithuania, France, and Bohemia as well. Military holy orders also began, populated by armed monks dedicated to the spread and protection of the Christian faith. In the thirteenth century, St Thomas Aquinas developed the "just war" theory that argued that Christians could go to war as long as the war was authorized by higher authority (meaning the Church and the king), was a means toward peace, and only contained violence proportionate to desired ends. Religion could thus limit warfare and its effects on non-combatants, but it could at the same time create a dichotomy of believers and non-believers that protected the former while demonizing the latter, often with brutal consequences.

Some of this era's most terrible battles occurred in northern India after the first appearance of Muslim armies there in 711. Those armies used a combination of horse and camel cavalry to push Hindu forces south and east. One war in the tenth century may have led to the destruction of as many as 10,000 Hindu temples. Religious and military motivations thus blended as a reflection of the increasing influence that world religions had on the world's peoples.

Third, most warriors in this period, especially in Europe and Japan, were tied to their lords by oaths of loyalty and obedience. These oaths were the products of the informal and decentralized political structures that replaced the classical civilizations. These structures, generally called feudalism, involved military and political obligations that bound knights to higher lords. In Europe, Charles Martel (714–741) is generally credited with creating this system out of land seized from church holdings.

In Japan a similar system evolved with the important difference that European feudalism was normally based on contractual obligations while the Japanese system was normally based on personal loyalty. In Japan the warrior classes and landed classes did not overlap as neatly as they did in the west. Rather, the system emerged from the constant state of civil war between rival Japanese clans.

The Japanese warriors, called samurai, were extremely skilled at riding, archery, and the expert use of the samurai's most important weapon, the sword. In this respect they resemble mounted warriors in the Middle East, Europe, and Mongol Asia. Samurai warfare, however, tended to be more highly ritualistic, with elaborate ceremonies and characterized by individual combat. The samurai understood failure on the battlefield as both a personal short-coming and a failure to honor the commitments made to their lord. Ritual suicide often followed a defeat. Unlike the European system, no formalized system existed to deal with prisoners because no honor was associated with the capture of a man who had failed in his obligations. Although they developed independently of one another, feudal systems across the global shared many key features. They created the foundations for the European and Japanese military aristocracies that developed in this period.

In contrast to Europe and Japan, Chinese civilization in the Middle Ages witnessed the domination of the civilian bureaucracy in military affairs, much to the detriment of the battlefield performance of Chinese forces. The emperors of the Song Dynasty (960 to 1279 CE), fearful that the military posed an internal threat to their rule, curtailed the traditional latitude of Chinese generals. As a result, although the armies of the Song were numerically large and technologically sophisticated, the Song had one of the worst military records of any Chinese dynasty up to that point. The armies of Song China suffered constant defeat at the hands of smaller and less well-equipped Central Asian nomads like the Mongols who eventually overthrew them.

Machines

The post-classical period is rarely associated with vast changes in military technology. Generally speaking, the weapons of infantrymen remained the same as they had for centuries: swords; spears; and bows. All were improved upon during this period, but a true paradigm shift in weapons systems would not come until the large-scale introduction of reliable gunpowder weapons in the fourteenth and fifteenth centuries.

The most important military technology of the period was not even a weapon. The iron stirrup, probably invented in India around 1 CE, did not come into general use until the eighth century in the Middle East. When it did come into general use, it defined the era. Like many technological systems of the post-classical era, it transferred quickly across civilization borders.

The production of iron stirrups and improvements in horse breeding allowed for the creation of a combined military system that some historians have likened to a post-classical version of the tank. In heavy cavalry units, a powerful war horse and rider were protected (or, depending on one's point of view, laden down) by as much as 100 pounds of armor. The stirrup allowed the rider to transfer the horse's power and speed into the thrust of a lance at his opponent's armor.

Alternatively, a rider could lighten his armor and use the horse's speed to quickly get into range and fire arrows from his bow. Mounted archery was not new, but stirrups made it a more powerful weapon. It proved to be more popular in the east because western nobles disdained the bow as a commoner's weapon. Bows became lighter and more powerful with the introduction of the composite bow, made from different strips of wood and other materials fused together to make a stronger final product than ancient bows fashioned from a single piece of wood. The composite bow and stirrup together allowed a skilled rider to shoot accurately and ride at the same time.

Swords played both a military and a ceremonial role. In close or dismounted combat, the sword became the mounted warrior's most important weapon. But the sword also had a tremendous role as a symbol of the social prestige and political power of its bearer, a role they continue today, long after they have lost any military value. Indeed, the knight's career began with a touch of a sword upon his shoulders.

A high-quality sword could take more than 200 hours of labor to fashion. In Japan, where swords were more important than they were anywhere else, sword makers dressed more like priests than laborers. In many places, only aristocrats and gentlemen could legally carry swords. In Japan, the right to carry two swords became an exclusive privilege of the samurai.

The sword was therefore a weapon of individual combat between peers. Other weapons threatened the very role of the gentleman on the battlefield. The crossbow, another technology developed in China that moved west, was one such weapon. It consisted of a wooden stock with a groove cut down the center into which the crossbowman placed an arrow or bolt. At the front was a large horn that, when an attached string was pulled back behind the arrow, provided the power. A pull of a trigger released the tension in the horn and dispatched the arrow.

Crossbowmen used a variety of arrows including pointed arrows designed to penetrate armor and flat ones designed to knock a knight off his horse. Although it had a slower rate of fire than normal bows, the crossbow's draw weight of more than 1,000 pounds provided significantly more power than conventional bows. The crossbow also required a much lower level of skill than traditional bows. Knights and samurai therefore reserved special disdain for crossbowmen. At the Lateran Council in 1139, the Catholic Church even banned its use against Christians. The ban made no attempt to prevent its use against non-Christians and, in the end, the ban was generally ignored anyway. Before the end of the twelfth century England's Richard the Lionhearted and France's Philip Augustus had both reintroduced the crossbow.

Perhaps the most famous technology of this period, and the one that is easiest to view firsthand today, is the castle. Castles served both as visible statements of an individual family's power and as a defensive work. Indeed, the continued existence of hundreds of post-classical castles across the world testify to their durability and importance. Large castles often included everything needed to withstand a long siege including gardens for growing fresh food, water storage tanks, and apothecaries.

Wealthy and frequently contested regions like Italy, Japan, and Palestine became heavily encastled as a way for lords to protect their wealth from rivals. By one count Norman nobles built 500 castles in England during the second half of the eleventh century alone. As the technology of castle construction evolved, so too did a parallel technology of siege warfare. A variety of siege engines existed, including a device called a trebuchet, which used a counter-weight system to throw a large stone accurately 200 yards or more. Mines and siege towers also made their appearance as did a primitive form of biological warfare; besieging forces would often dump dead animals into their opponents' moats or catapult them over walls in an effort to destroy the water supply and generate disease.

In 1131 a Syrian knight named Usamah Ibn-Munqidh took part in the siege of the Crusader castle of Kafartab. He describes the extensive Islamic efforts to take the castle, especially the tunnels constructed to undermine the stronghold from below:

> I went down in the trench, while the arrows and stones were falling on us like rain, and entered the tunnel. There I was struck with the great wisdom with which the digging was executed. The tunnel was dug from the trench to the barbican. On the sides of the tunnel were set up two pillars, across which stretched a plank to prevent the earth above it from falling down. The whole tunnel had such a framework of wood that extended as far as the foundation of the [enemy] tower. The tunnel was narrow. It was nothing but a means to provide access to the tower. As soon as they got to the tower, they enlarged the tunnel in[to] the wall of the tower, supported it on timbers and began to carry out, a little at a time, the splinters of stone produced by boring.[1]

By such tedious and difficult work in the height of a summer sun, the Islamic armies caused the tower to collapse, took the castle, and won the battle.

Castles protected the residences of lords; larger fortifications protected entire cities. Using architectural methods similar to those used by castle designers, engineers constructed elaborate defensive works. The fortifications at Constantinople were among the world's most powerful, including a double wall 100 feet wide and a powerful chain that stretched across the Golden Horn to stop shipping. Not all fortifications were as powerful, but virtually all places of any military importance in the world were protected by walls, towers, moats, and other features. Although the Japanese and European fortification styles shared many features in common, it is extremely unlikely that they influenced one another. Instead, their designs were common responses to the decentralized nature of politics in the post-classical period.

At the end of the post-classical period, the introduction of primitive gunpowder weapons finally undid the knight's dominance. But one other weapon foreshadowed that end: the longbow. First used as a hunting weapon in England and Wales, by the thirteenth century English kings began to introduce longbows into their armies. The longbow, as its name implies, was a large as six feet long and, in the hands of a skilled archer, proved deadly. The longer string and bow allowed for greater killing power. Its effective range was as long as 200 yards and it could fire about five times as quickly as a crossbow. For these reasons, England abandoned the crossbow by the middle of the fourteenth century in favor of the longbow.

The results were dramatic. In 1346 at the Battle of Crécy and again at Poitiers in 1356, English longbowmen (who needed years of practice to master their weapon) used their superior rate of fire to dispatch Italian mercenary crossbowmen in the service of the French army. They then turned on French knights, who were defenseless in the face of a rain of arrows. Although few realized it at the time (the French certainly did not), Crécy and Poitiers marked a great turning point in the military relationship between infantry and cavalry. French failure to adapt cost them another terrible defeat at the hands of the new weapon in 1415. Almost 5,000 French knights died in one day at the Battle of Agincourt that year. In a battle made famous by Shakespeare in his *Henry V*, longbowmen in the English army withered slowly advancing French cavalry.

The machines of the post-classical period reflected the dominant political and social patterns of the period. In the beginning of the period, the system was based around the individual aristocratic knight, armed with exquisite swords and protected by expensive armor and castles. Commoners had little military role other than the production of the wealth the lord needed. As the period developed, however, warlords looked for ways to undermine the power of the mounted warrior. They found their answer in hand-held weapons that could be used by commoners. Bows, and eventually, guns, ended the age of the feudal knight, returning infantry to the place of primacy on the battlefield.

The battles

Many of the wars of this period reflect one or all of the main themes of the period discussed above: the general dominance of mounted warriors; the role of religion as a motivating factor; and the political decentralization of this period as the western Roman, Gupta, and Han Empires ebbed. To cite just one example, Rome was attacked eight separate times and taken six times between 410 and 563.

Because strong centralized governments were rarer in this period than in the previous period, the post-classical period witnessed many raids. The widely feared Vikings used longboats and cavalry to appear with little warning and plunder unprepared victims. Viking ships could carry as many as sixty-four men and had a low draught, allowing them to easily beach, raid, then leave as quickly as they came. Raids at festival times, when wealth was particularly concentrated, were common. Their fearsome reputation, especially for plundering towns that had resisted them, led many villages to agree to whatever extortion demand the Vikings made.

With one of the most powerful of the post-classical military systems, the Mongols took great advantage of the collapse of the centralized classical civilizations by pushing into China, Russia, Korea, and the Caucasus. By the early thirteenth century Genghis Khan had united rival Mongol tribes into a potent force that used compound bows and fast, light cavalry to achieve military supremacy. With a population of about 1,500,000 they subdued and conquered communities much larger than their own.

Their ferocity soon earned them the same well-deserved reputation for military prowess that the Vikings also possessed. Concepts like Japanese *bushido*, Chinese *li* and western chivalry did not exist in the Mongol world. For the Mongols a reputation for ferocity served them well. The mere appearance of a Mongol army was often enough to induce towns to surrender. To enhance their reputation, the Mongols sometimes killed all adult males from a conquered tribe and took adult women and children, incorporating them into Mongol families. When the Mongols overthrew the Abbasid Caliphate in Baghdad in 1258 they killed 500,000 people and stacked their hearts in a pyramid to deter further resistance. They also rolled the last Abbasid Caliph in a carpet and ran their horses over him.

Basing a system on mounted warriors, no matter how good, had disadvantages as well. Because their system was based on speed, the Mongols were not as good as Europeans at siege warfare. Unless the Mongols could find Chinese engineers to conduct sieges, they had a difficult time capturing heavily-defended cities. They also could not conduct operations in geographical areas that could not provide horse fodder, such as the deserts of Syria or the jungles of southeast Asia. Two massive naval expeditions against Japan in 1274 and 1281 also failed. The 1281 expedition involved an astonishing 150,000 warriors, slightly larger than the number of allied troops landed on the first day of the invasion of France in 1944 discussed in the introduction. Despite these shortcomings, the Mongols dominated the age of cavalry, subjugating those areas where they could effectively use their superior horses and horsemen.

The Mongol overthrow of the Song Dynasty in 1279 further proves the dominance of cavalry over infantry that we have seen in the Middle East and Europe as well. The Song had superior numbers and technology, including primitive gas, gunpowder, and flame-based weapons, but their army was almost entirely infantry. The Chinese could not overcome the speed and mobility that Mongol cavalry provided. Mongol horsemen could converge on a given point, a tactic they practiced often, yielding a temporary advantage in numbers at that point and making the Chinese believe that the Mongol forces were much larger than in fact they were.

Chinese and Mongol warfare generally lacked faith-based justifications. Elsewhere, religion proved to be critical. European and Indian efforts to stem the rising tide of Islam formed the center of many important battles in this era. Christian armies turned back the Moors in France at the Battle of Tours in 732. Charles Martel used cavalry in equal numbers with infantry to drive the Muslim forces back into Spain. At the key moment of Muslim attack, Martel ordered his cavalry to dismount and form a solid phalanx. It is not clear from surviving records how many Frankish warriors were using stirrups; a lack of stirrups may have compelled Martel to order his men off their horses, where they would have been at a significant disadvantage. The Franks in any case resisted a strong Muslim charge and the seemingly irresistible tide of Islam had finally been turned back, though it had not been eliminated. Christian armies fought until the end of the fifteenth century to reconquer Spain.

Tours represents the western end of Christian-Muslim warfare. Fighting in the Middle East also pitted Christians against Muslims. The eight Crusades called by the west between 1095 and 1291 show the overlap of the three themes discussed above. In the First Crusade, 30,000 non-noble Christians volunteered to fight, motivated in part by papal promises that their sins would be absolved. Lacking armor or training, 25,000 of them were slaughtered by the Turks. Future crusades were therefore noble-led operations, inspired both by papal desires to recapture the Holy Land from the Muslims and noble desires to enrich themselves. Kings and lords used a combination of religious appeal and feudal obligation to entice knights to undertake crusades. In the Third Crusade, King Richard the Lionhearted of England, Philip Augustus of France, and Holy Roman Emperor Frederick Barbarossa all crusaded personally and brought along their personal vassals.

The Crusades revealed the same discrepancy between western and eastern warfare that was demonstrated at Manzikert. Western knights tended to be slow, heavily armored, and preferred hand-to-hand weapons like lances and swords. Muslim armies tended toward light cavalry constituted of mobile archers. As at Manzikert (and throughout most of the Middle East), the advantage lay with light cavalry. Muslim armies grew even stronger after their superior cavalry handed the Mongols their first major defeat at the Battle of Ayn Jalut in the deserts of Palestine in 1260. Thereafter, the Muslims did not need to worry about the approaching Mongols and could focus on the Christians.

Because mounted warriors could not easily take a castle, siege warfare grew increasingly more complex during this period. Essentially, a siege involves cutting a castle or fort off from external resupply until it is compelled by hunger or thirst to surrender. Sieges are as old as that of Jericho (believed to have taken place in 1350 BCE), but the proliferation of defensive works made them much more common in this period.

Sieges tended to be among the nastiest and bloodiest form of warfare because of the human costs involved in storming defenses, and because commonly-recognized international law permitted the killing or enslavement of those who refused to surrender. Furthermore, the more nastily an army treated the survivors of a siege, the less likely future enemies might be to resist. The Manchus, the Mongols, and some crusaders were well known for their cruel sieges. The Christians slaughtered all inhabitants of Antioch in 1098 and Jerusalem in 1099. This strategy backfired when inhabitants so feared their besiegers that they held out all the more fervently. Such people tried to hold out as long as absolutely possible in the hopes that either the besiegers would give up or help might arrive. Sieges of heavily provisioned areas could therefore last for years.

Another way to entice an armed force out of its castle was to devastate its hinterland. Organized raids, called *chevauchées* in Europe, both enriched those doing the plundering and forced opposing armies to risk battle. *Chevauchées* laid waste to miles and miles of territory, without distinguishing between military and civilian targets. They could be a major impetus toward forcing one's enemies to ask for peace, but they could also produce enmity for decades.

The series of wars collectively known as the Hundred Years War between England and France (1337 to 1453) shows the conflicting and chaotic nature of European feudalism. Because noble families often inter-married and because vassals often accepted land from several lords, patterns of European feudal loyalty and succession were always in doubt. When French king Charles V died without a male heir in 1328, the English king Edward III used an old feudal claim to declare himself king of France. Edward was both king of England and duke of Aquitaine, in southwestern France. Three of Edward's uncles had sat on the French throne. Still, French knights refused to accept the union of their fiefdoms under a fifteen-year old English king. Both sides thus had to cajole, bribe, and enforce feudal dues in order to procure enough knights to fight the war.

As noted above, English longbowmen devastated French knights in several battles during the Hundred Years War. At Crécy in 1346 English longbowmen devastated a French force nearly three times larger than their own. Slow-moving knights especially suffered. The French lost 1,542 lords and knights at Crécy; the English lost just two men of equivalent stature. Similar disasters awaited French knights at Poitiers in 1356 where 2,500 died and an equal number more became prisoners. The slaughter at Agincourt (1415) added 5,000 more dead knights. English financial problems and the appearance of the charismatic Joan of Arc in 1428 enabled France to emerge victorious, but the longbow presented French mounted knights with an obvious challenge that they never fully addressed.

The steady decline of the power of the knight combined with the growing expense of warfare inevitably produced pressures for change. In 1340 the cost of wages alone for the English army stood at £60,000 at a time when total royal revenues equaled only £40,000. Kings and dukes began to look for ways to control the chaotic, undisciplined, and costly feudal system. By the fourteenth century the Italians had introduced a more commercial and contractual military system in an attempt to control the growing chaos and expenses. These contractual soldiers, called *condottieri*, laid the foundation both for the development of national armies and the expansion of professional mercenaries.

Legacies

The dominance of cavalry, light and heavy, is the most important similarity between eastern and western warfare in the post-classical period. Improved horse-breeding and technologies like the stirrup produced a distinct advantage to the mounted warrior. Classical infantry weapons like swords and simple bows could not compensate for the speed and power of cavalry. By the end of this period the crossbow and the longbow had begun to tip the scales, but gunpowder weapons, to be discussed in Chapter 3, finally changed the relationship between infantry and cavalry.

Therefore, those systems that relied too heavily on infantry often lost to those that adequately incorporated horses and camels. The success of Islamic forces, the Mongols, and the Seljuk Turks, all of whom used cavalry effectively, demonstrates the power of mounted warfare. The inability of Late Song China, the Byzantines, and others to handle mounted warriors graphically proves the point as well.

Today's armies look more like the infantry-based armies of the classical period than the cavalry-based armies of the post-classical period. Modern militaries share their emphasis on mass (sometimes citizen) armies with the ancients, not with the more exclusive and aristocratic systems of the post-classical centuries. Still, it took several centuries for cavalry to lose the mystique and prestige that it acquired in the post-classical period. Although in most armies cavalry moved from the center to one element of a combined arms force, the sublime image of the horse stayed in the minds of military men for centuries. As late as 1925, Field Marshal Sir Douglas Haig, commander of British forces in World War I, argued that well-bred horses were still the military equal to planes, tanks, and armored vehicles.

Religion played a much more central role in warfare in western Europe and the Middle East than it did in East Asia. The religious hatreds stirred up in this period have yet to completely fade. Modern crises between Pakistan and India as well as those between western governments and Middle Eastern ones have significant historical roots in this period. Memories of the Crusades took a long time to fade for both Christians and Muslims. Warfare between religious groups was, of course, not limited to this period. As we will see, the dichotomies and antagonisms of the post-classical period continued to serve as root and proximate causes of warfare.

Note

1 Quoted in John Keegan, *The Book of War* (New York: Viking, 1999), pp. 43–44.

Further reading

Maurice Keen, ed. *Medieval Warfare: A History* (Oxford: Oxford University Press, 1999) is an excellent place to begin; see also his *Laws of War in the Late Middle Ages* (London: Routledge, 1965) as well as Malcolm Vale, *War and Chivalry* (Cambridge: Cambridge University Press, 1996). For a readable account of the Mongols, see David Morgan, *The Mongols* (Cambridge, Mass.: Blackwell, 1990). For the Crusades, start with Jonathan Riley-Smith, *The Crusades: A Short History* (New Haven: Yale University Press, 1987) and R. C. Smail, *Crusading Warfare, 1097–1193* (Cambridge: Cambridge University Press, 1956). For Agincourt, see the relevant chapter in John Keegan, *The Face of Battle* (New York: Viking Press, 1976). For the Samurai see Stephen Turnbull, *Samurai Warfare* (New York: Sterling Press, 1996). See also Kelly DeVries, *Infantry Warfare in the Early 14th Century: Discipline, Tactics, and Technology* (Rochester, NY: Boydell Press, 1996) and John France, *Western Warfare in the Age of the Crusades, 1000–1300* (Ithaca: Cornell University Press, 1999).

Chapter 3

The emergence of gunpowder weapons, 1450 to 1776

Québec, 1759

Throughout the sixteenth, seventeenth, and eighteenth centuries, European armies and navies had endeavored to create global empires. Their powerful ships and guns gave them tremendous advantages over Asian, African, and American peoples who lacked such technology. As the empires grew, they inevitably began to collide with one another. By the middle of the eighteenth century the British and French empires were encroaching upon one another across the globe. When war broke out in Europe in 1756, it soon spread to colonial outposts from India to Canada.

British general James Wolfe, a middle-class professional officer, led an army against the city of Québec, the key to French Canada. Wolfe had recently commanded successful expeditions against French garrisons in Nova Scotia, Acadia, and Louisbourg, the island fortress that guarded the entry to the St Lawrence Seaway. He knew that the powerful English navy could deny the French garrison resupply by sea. Wolfe still had to overcome a powerful French fort, the Citadelle, that protected the city and defeat an experienced French commander, the Marquis de Montcalm.

Wolfe was outnumbered 15,000 to 9,000. His men were, however, mostly highly-trained professionals. Montcalm, on the other hand, had to rely primarily on militia because Britain's Royal Navy prevented reinforcements of French regulars from reaching Québec. Wolfe's great problem was scaling the cliffs near the city and landing his men on the Plains of Abraham, a thousand-yard wide, rolling plain that sat outside the Citadelle. If he could find a way to do so, he could cut the French off from land as they had already been cut off from sea.

Wolfe's opportunity came when deserters told him that the French were expecting supplies to arrive by ship on the night of 12 September at a point two miles south of the city. Wolfe sent a detachment to pose as the supply party, then get ashore. Most of his army followed, while a smaller portion held to the north of the city to create a diversion. By dawn, he had 4,800 men on the Plains of Abraham marching toward the city. Montcalm, stunned that

Wolfe had outfoxed him, had a difficult decision to make. He could surely withdraw to the Citadelle and withstand any British attack, but doing so would cut him off from vital land supply routes just as the brutal Canadian winter was ready to begin. He therefore chose to lead his inferior militia out of the fortress and engage the British.

Montcalm's militia, less well-trained in close order drill and tactics, fired from 130 yards, too far to be effective. Wolfe's men, professional and experienced, knew that they could lie down at the instant that the French shot because Montcalm had no cavalry to charge at them. After firing his volley, Montcalm saw no choice but to order his men forward with bayonets. The British waited for the French to get within forty yards, then took their turn; their lethal volley killed 500 French soldiers. The French militia panicked and returned to the safety of the Citadelle. Among the 500 dead was Montcalm; the British had lost just fifty-eight men, including Wolfe. Once inside the Citadelle, the demoralized and leaderless French garrison faced a grim situation. Without French infantry on the plains, the British were free to bring up cannon and begin a winter siege. The French surrendered Québec less than a week later. French rule in Canada had been dealt a severe blow by a single volley delivered by professional musketeers.

Québec displays several of the dominant changes of this age. First, the power of gunpowder weapons in the hands of trained professionals was perfectly evident in this period; thus it is often called simply "the gunpowder age." Those armies that could match the latest technologies with men capable of producing and using them enjoyed tremendous advantages. Second, navies took on unprecedented importance as colonies became more central to the economic life of mother countries. Here Great Britain took a lead that it would hold until World War II. Finally, this period reflects the growing importance of dynastic motivations as gunpowder facilitated the centralization of power and the growing strength of monarchy.

The men

The military history of this period must necessarily focus on the revolution brought about by gunpowder weapons. Nevertheless, keep in mind that the introduction of new weapons systems always depends on the right social, cultural, political, and economic environments. In some parts of the world, notably East Asia and the Middle East, these environments proved unfriendly to the adaptation of gunpowder weapons. In Europe, by contrast, the environment proved much more receptive. Europe's more rapid incorporation of guns should be read not as evidence of European superiority but as a function of key elements of the European environment, including: constant warfare (Europe was in a state of total peace for only ten years between 1500 and 1700); relatively open free enterprise system; political instability; and availability of key natural resources like coal and iron.

As we saw in the previous chapter, the power of aristocratic mounted warriors was waning even before gunpowder weapons came to dominate the battlefield. In the place of armies centered around mounted knights emerged dynastic armies centrally controlled by kings and, in some cases, parliaments. In contrast to Japan and the Middle East, then, European aristocrats were in a weaker position to resist changes in the nature of warfare. Japanese samurai and Islamic mamluks were better able to use their power to effectively marginalize gunpowder weapons because of the threat that such weapons posed to their monopoly on military power.

Because aristocrats initially tended to disdain gunpowder weapons, many European kings turned to mercenaries (foreigners who served primarily for money) to man armies. Although they were relatively expensive, mercenaries came already trained in the latest weapons systems and did not require a prince to undertake the unpopular step of demanding military service from his own people. When regularly paid, mercenaries provided a highly-skilled and reliable way of manning an army. The great disadvantage of mercenaries was their focus on money. They might refuse to fight at a crucial time or they might demand more money than had been previously agreed to. If their payment was slow in coming, they might turn on their employer. They frequently ravaged and looted, often without regard for their victims' ostensible allegiance. Kings therefore began to seek ways to obtain loyalty from another source.

In the sixteenth century Charles V's Spain led the way in creating permanent regiments with their own uniforms, traditions, and group loyalties. Over time, these regiments, called *tercios*, produced their own uniforms and insignia to further distinguish them from other units. Such regiments attracted men who genuinely sought the camaraderie and martial spirit that military service provided. Militaries motivated by regimental loyalty often translated that élan into greater spirit and efficiency on the battlefield. From these beginnings emerged the permanent regiments that continue to characterize modern armies today. Ideally, these units were constituted of national soldiers, loyal both to their unit and their homeland. In reality, mercenaries often filled the ranks of regiments because national loyalty remained low in many regions and because military service carried with it little prestige or chance at social betterment.

Military service at the enlisted level did not carry much prestige because mass armies based around gunpowder weapons reduced the overall skill level of military service. Because almost any man could use gunpowder weapons if properly trained, guns put emphasis on rigid discipline rather than on skill at arms. To fire gunpowder weapons effectively in volleys required getting men to complete the requisite series of steps in concert. Maurice of Nassau, the Dutch prince who in the early seventeenth century created modern drill tactics, believed that only intense discipline could transform men into reliable instruments of state policy. His ideas caught on across Europe. The result for soldiers was a life of constant, and often capricious, discipline. In many armies men feared their own officers more than they feared the enemy.

In 1607, Maurice introduced the first modern drill manuals to create uniform discipline standards and tactical capabilities among his men. He also experimented with tactical formations to get the most from his men. Maurice and his most important disciple, King Gustavus Adolphus of Sweden, developed the linear formation. Musketeers lined up in rows, normally six to ten men deep. The first line fired its volley, then retreated to the back to reload while the second line advanced. If men could be trained to continue this system in an orderly fashion under hostile fire, an army could keep up a nearly continuous rate of fire. The Thirty Years War (1618–1648) proved the deadly effectiveness of this system.

Chinese general Ch'i Chi-kuang reintroduced drill in China at about the same time that Maurice was redefining drill in Europe. Chinese armies generally made less use of gunpowder weapons than did western ones, but the Chinese may well have emphasized drill because of a belief in drill's ability to forge esprit de corps and promote action in unison. As a result of constant drill and discipline, the quality of life in an army regiment could be extremely unpleasant and most men avoided it if at all possible.

The Chinese proverb "Good iron is not used to make nails; good men are not used to make soldiers" sums up the attitude of many civilians toward common soldiers and sailors. The stereotypical soldier of this period joined out of dire financial need. Sometimes military service came in lieu of, or addition to, a criminal sentence. For many poor peasants, the military served as an employer of last resort or a way for men to escape from problems in their home villages. Recruiters' jobs were usually easiest in times of high food prices and economic recession. Only in highly-skilled areas like gunnery and engineering did military service lend much prestige. These jobs came to be dominated by members of the middle class such as James Wolfe because the bourgeoisie was the only group in Europe with the requisite skills necessary to handle the complex tasks involved.

Mass armies also posed an obvious threat to the social status of military elites. Not surprisingly, then, European knights, Islamic mamluks, and Japanese samurai often tried to slow or prevent the introduction of gunpowder weapons. Only in Japan did they fully succeed. After a brief period of experimenting with guns, which they learned about from the Portuguese, the Japanese effectively banned guns in the seventeenth century as part of a more general process of reducing or eliminating foreign influences. The Japanese case proves the point that the mere existence of guns did not suffice to change closely held and cherished societal beliefs. A society could, and in this case certainly did, learn about guns, master their use, then decide to give them up. The samurai thereby held onto their exalted position in Japanese society until the mid-nineteenth century.

Although the European aristocracy's monopoly on military power dissolved, nobles continued to play a military role through dominance of the prestigious officer corps; hence Montcalm's command at Québec. Because of the system of primogeniture, eldest sons inherited titles, money, and land, leaving younger sons with no evident role. As a result, many became military officers. The word "cadet" comes from the French word for youngest son. Some sons obtained their commissions through purchasing them. Other officers, like the famous British general John Churchill, were born into minor, and often impoverished, gentry families. Military service provided a means of social advancement. For his service to the English kings, Churchill became the Duke of Marlborough at the age of fifty-two. Like many officers of this period, he used his military service to compensate for the poverty of his family.

The expense of warfare also led to increasing centralization of military administration. France's growing power in Europe after the middle of the seventeenth century owed much to the increasing power of the French monarchy under Louis XIV and the efficient administration of men like Louis' finance minister Jean Baptiste Colbert, who always found ways to fund the king's costly wars. France also created a virtual army of minor bureaucrats and functionaries who handled the daily tasks of running an army. These reforms provided a more regular efficiency and stability than had previously existed in European militaries.

Military reforms reflected a larger complexity of organizational changes. This period witnessed the first modern pensions and hospitals, sparing old veterans the humiliation of having to beg at convents or in the streets. In 1670 France founded the most famous of these early facilities, Paris' beautiful gold-domed Hôtel des Invalides, capable of caring for 4,000 men in grandeur and dignity. As a mark of the building's importance, Napoleon's body was entombed there in 1840.

As was the case in European politics and economics, military administration centralized. Oliver Cromwell's New Model Army, introduced in 1645, imposed a common model on all British militia and regular troops. Cromwell introduced the famous British redcoat uniform and forced local militia to accept service in campaigns beyond their home territories. Although these reforms generated significant opposition, they gave the British a true professional military force.

One other, very different, model for manning an army existed in the Islamic world. Turkish sultans used slave soldiers, called janissaries. Because the Koran forbids the enslavement of Muslims, the sultans sent representatives to scour the countryside in search of non-Muslim (usually Christian) boys aged eight to eighteen. The boys took on Muslim names, trained intensively, and led a nearly monastic lifestyle. They accepted lifelong military service in exchange for wealth and the promise of a special place in heaven. By many accounts, they were the most feared and respected soldiers in the world in the fifteenth and sixteenth centuries. A force of 10,000 janissaries was an integral component of Sultan Mehmet II's capture of Constantinople in 1453. The janissaries grew wealthy from the loot and plunder they took from the city as their reward.

The machines

Gunpowder weapons dominated this era. Although gunpowder had been known in China since at least the ninth century, it was not until the fifteenth century that gunpowder weapons came into general use. One reason for the delay was the unreliability of propellants. Until the 1420 discovery of the process of "corning" (rolling and dampening) gunpowder, the substance's extreme volatility made it as much a danger to the user as the intended victim. For years afterward, gunpowder weapons took as much courage to use as to face in battle. In 1460 Scotland's James II became one of the famous commanders killed by one of his own malfunctioning guns.

Although gunpowder itself was first developed in Asia, Europe excelled in the construction of guns. On the economic level, Europe's free enterprise and banking systems provided financial incentives and relative freedom to gunsmiths to innovate. The ability of Europeans to cast large church bells ironically converted into an ability to cast guns. Making guns from a single cast proved to be much stronger than fusing together individual pieces of metal; the gun that accidentally killed James II had been fused. Furthermore, the near-constant nature of European warfare gave princes an incentive to fund research and entrepreneurs a ready market for new weapons systems.

Two kinds of guns existed: small arms, capable of being used by an individual, and siege guns (artillery), so large that they sometimes had to be cast on site. The latter proved their battlefield efficacy first, as early as the 1370s. By 1450 one such gun, "Mons Meg," still on display at Edinburgh Castle in Scotland, was fifteen feet long, weighed fifteen tons, and fired an eighteen-inch projectile, usually made of stone. In 1453, Ottoman Turkish armies used similarly massive guns, called bombards, to decimate Constantinople's once-formidable defenses. The Sultan's seventy large guns reputedly included one that had a twenty-six foot barrel. Constantinople's walls, which for centuries had withstood sieges by Persians, Huns, Magyars, Arabs, Berbers, Tartars, and Turks, fell in just six weeks. The world's castles and fortifications, with their high walls and towers, soon became anachronisms.

By the middle of the sixteenth century, a wide variety of iron, brass, and bronze guns had emerged. Wealthy states like Spain led the way with large guns called culverins that could fire thirty-two pound projectiles as far as 7,000 yards. The warring Italian city-states also became a center of gun innovation. Among these new weapons were mortars, designed to fire projectiles at high trajectories to fly over fortifications and walls. By the time of the Thirty Years War European guns were smaller and more mobile, allowing truly effective field artillery to play a role on the battlefield other than scaring horses.

Reliable small arms developed around the same time. The first useful gun, the arquebus, was so heavy that it had to be rested on a wooden fork. It was fired by the application of a match to gunpowder in a pan. A later development, the matchlock, was fired through the use of an "S" shaped device called a serpentine. The serpentine held a smoldering or burning match that, when released by a trigger, ignited the gunpowder. The range of this weapon was considerably shorter than that of a longbow (no more than eighty to 100 yards) and its rate of fire was much slower, but guns could do far more damage to men and armor, especially at close range.

Early small arms were notoriously inaccurate, so inaccurate in fact, that men normally fired in large volleys without aiming. The standard command was "ready, level, fire." "Ready, aim, fire" came later. But as technology improved, so did the performance of small arms. Over time, specially cast iron balls replaced stones as ammunition and the quality of the guns themselves improved. Matchlocks improved the reliability of guns, but their burning wicks were still vulnerable to wind and rain. In the middle of the sixteenth century, a German inventor developed the flintlock, which partially solved the problem of weather. The flintlock, as its name implies, operates by the strike of flint upon steel. The ensuing sparks ignited the powder and stood up better to wind and light rain.

With the development of the flintlock, a true infantry weapon had appeared. The invention of the ring bayonet in the 1690s allowed the infantryman to defend himself against cavalry and infantry charges between volleys. Still, the expense, inaccuracy, and slow fire rate of guns meant that their introduction took time. England did not give up the longbow until 1595 and even as late as the American Revolution many people, Benjamin Franklin among them, argued for the longbow as the colonists' main infantry weapon.

Reservations notwithstanding, the advantages of guns were obvious to most. But keeping one's arsenal up to date was an extremely costly venture that only the very wealthiest states could afford. The balance of power in the world thus shifted in favor of those who could afford the new guns and the new fortifications required to counter the guns. The power of kings and emperors therefore grew in relation to that of minor nobles. The new "gunpowder empires" included England, Spain, and France in western Europe, the Moguls in India, the Ottomans in the Middle East, Czarist Russia in eastern Europe, and, in a different fashion, the Ch'ing (Manchus) in China. These empires used gunpowder weapons and centralized administrations to expand at the expense of neighboring principalities.

Wealthy empires had the resources to update their guns continually and meet the challenge of redesigning their fortifications. Older fortifications, such as those at Constantinople, were vulnerable to guns. Their high walls could be easily attacked by artillery fire aimed at the base. New fortifications, like the Citadelle at Québec, contained parallel lines of lower, angled walls to deflect cannon balls and packed earth to absorb their shock. Among the most effective were those designed in the seventeenth century by France's famous engineer, Sébastien Le Prestre de Vauban, which employed artillery towers, ramparts, and geometrical designs to create interlocking fields of fire. Vauban believed that basing warfare around fortifications would spare the lives of innocent civilians caught between campaigning armies. Several of the best fortifications from this period remained effective until World War I.

Moving field artillery pieces proved to be exceptionally difficult. The guns and requisite trains of ammunition were simply too cumbersome to move easily across broken terrain. Europeans could, however, take advantage of their large multi-sail ships, designed for the rough seas of the Atlantic Ocean. By cutting gun ports in their hulls, Europeans could turn their navies into powerful weapons. The largest naval battle of this period, the Battle of Lepanto, fought off the western coast of Greece in 1571, demonstrated the power of naval gunnery. A combined Spanish and Venetian fleet, though outnumbered in ships, used its 1,815 to 750 advantage in guns to destroy 200 of the Turkish fleet's 230 galleys.

Control of the seas therefore became a fundamental concern for states. The dominance of Spanish fleets in the sixteenth century helps to account for that empire's wealth. Not to be outdone, England's Protestant King Henry VIII used funds from seized Catholic Church lands to build a powerful fleet that, after the 1588 defeat of the Spanish Armada, gave England command of the seas. After that battle, where superior English guns proved their worth, England became the world's most powerful naval force. In 1759, England built the revolutionary HMS Victory, a warship with no equal. It required sixty acres worth of wood from oak trees, twenty-seven miles of rope, and four acres of sails to construct. Its three gun decks contained 104 guns of four sizes. In the hands of an expert crew it could fire a broadside of 1,100 pounds of iron every ninety seconds.

Throughout this period, European technology grew by leaps and bounds in comparison to that of other regions. The Ottomans continued to build on their success at Constantinople at 1453 but viewed gunpowder weapons largely as long-range battering rams. China preferred not to experiment too much with the new technologies for fear of disrupting the Confucian order of society and state. They also chose not to develop the strong naval vessels that Europeans used to make their guns mobile. Furthermore, Asian and Muslim military elites like the Egyptian mamluks, Ottoman janissaries, and Japanese samurai proved to be more successful in resisting guns than their western European counterparts. As a result, Europe dominated the new military technologies and, through them, began to realize a vital advantage on the battlefield and on the high seas.

The battles

Those societies that could effectively incorporate gunpowder weapons and associated discipline and tactics into their military systems were at a distinct advantage over those that could not. Nowhere was this pattern more evident than in the Spanish conquest of the Americas in the sixteenth century. Aztec warriors commonly carried weapons designed to disable their opponents. The Aztecs placed great value on capturing human sacrifices as part of religious ceremonies. Some Amerindian groups used bronze arrows that proved to be deadly in combat, but no American weapon could consistently match Spanish firepower. Guns were not the only cause of the Spanish conquest (smallpox and other diseases killed many times more Amerindians than guns did), but their military and psychological value should not be underestimated. The English, Dutch, Portuguese, and French used similar technological advantages to create empires of their own in the Americas at the expense of native peoples who lacked guns.

Furthermore, Europeans brought to the Americas an understanding of warfare that had been conditioned by centuries of internecine struggles. Descended from Greek and Roman concepts of warfare, Europeans brought with them a definition of combat that stressed killing, not capture. This understanding of war as a pitched, brutal struggle was just as important as the technological advantages that Europeans held over their American (as well as Asian and African) enemies.

In Asia, the success of Muslim ruler Babur's invasion of northern India also owed much to his incorporation of Ottoman guns. In 1525 and 1526 he pushed across the Punjab and seized Delhi, establishing the Mogul Empire. Babur's grandson, Akbar the Great, used artillery and musketeers to create a powerful "gunpowder empire" similar in broad outline to those of his European contemporaries like Elizabeth I of England and Charles V of Spain.

But it was in Europe that guns most radically altered the nature of warfare. The most important European war of this period mixed dynastic and religious motivations. The Thirty Years War began as a struggle between Catholics and Protestants (themselves bitterly divided between Calvinists and Lutherans) for control of the principalities in what is now Germany. Because the states of Europe had invested so much money in guns and the training of dynastic armies, the war unleashed the full military and religious energies of Europe. Soon, virtually every army in Europe was engaged. The original religious motivations blurred as states vied to gain at the expense of their neighbors. Catholic Spain and Catholic France (the latter allied to Protestant Sweden and Holland) fought one another fiercely.

The Thirty Years War confirmed the supremacy of the new technologies and the new military systems that had evolved to manage them. Armies, like the Swedish armies commanded by Gustavus Adolphus, that featured disciplined troops with an effective combination of small arms and artillery, defeated those that had yet to master the new system. At the Battle of Breitenfeld in Saxony in 1631, Gustavus's disciplined Swedish army (which was three-quarters mercenary) defeated John Tserclaes von Tilly's army of the Holy Roman Empire through excellent field discipline and superior firepower. Gustavus's fifty-one to twenty-seven edge in field guns proved to be advantageous.

The presence of mercenary armies in the Thirty Years War caused terrible dislocations. By one estimate, as many as 1,000,000 men served during the course of the war. Because regular payments often failed to reach armies in the field, mercenaries and other soldiers often turned to looting and pillaging. The German principalities were almost helpless to resist the converging armies. Entire villages were wiped out. One German city changed hands eighteen times in two years, and was pillaged every time. The city of Mainz lost twenty-five per cent of its dwellings, forty per cent of its population, and sixty per cent of its total wealth.

The proliferation of modern weapons in the hands of trained mercenaries combined with religious fervor created a war whose horrors stunned contemporaries. Most modern sources estimate that the Thirty Years War killed over 7,000,000 civilians. The loss of life in many parts of Europe, especially Germany, was proportionately greater than during World War II. The horrors of the Thirty Years War and the equal horrors of the English Civil War (1642–1648) caused Europeans to look for ways to limit and minimize warfare.

The onset of the Enlightenment led to further considerations on the place of warfare in an "enlightened" age. Rationality was to be extended even to the battlefield; armies motivated by ideology or religious fervor came to be seen as irrational and therefore dangerous. Several important generals of this period argued that one should win battles by maneuver and diplomacy rather than by extended killing. This type of thinking led to the ideas of men like Vauban who hoped to isolate civilians from warfare by focusing combat on sieges and fortifications.

Technology also contributed to the search for limits to warfare. As the new weapons became more mature they also became more costly in human terms. Offensive charges and attacks against field artillery and effective small arms like flintlocks therefore came to be seen as wasteful. In the 1709 Battle of Malplaquet, direct charges against musketeers led to 36,000 casualties in just seven hours. Under the command of the Duke of Marlborough, England, though victorious, still lost twenty-five per cent of its army in one afternoon. Losses such as these were so disproportionate to desired state aims that European monarchs began to move away from pitched battle.

European states began therefore to fight "limited wars" for limited gains and at limited expense. Armies no longer sought to eliminate their foes. Instead they fought for precise state aims. Wars became less costly and warfare itself became an instrument for European diplomats. Gains and losses on the battlefield became trading pieces for statesmen to barter. For example, during King George's War (1743–1748), England seized the strategic French fortress of Louisbourg, at the mouth of the St Lawrence Seaway in Canada. English diplomats later gave the fortress back to the French in exchange for a French outpost halfway around the world in Madras, India. Louisbourg therefore had to be retaken by the English in a future war.

The battlefield in Europe at this time tended to be formal, tightly controlled by officers and NCOs. Maneuvers tended to be carefully choreographed and precisely timed. Prussia's Frederick the Great won a decisive battle at Leuthen in 1757 by quickly and effectively marching his men behind hills and trees then, at exactly the right moment, moving them rapidly from marching column to fighting line. Only perfectly disciplined troops could have completed such a move. The victory reinforced Frederick's sterling reputation as a great commander and made Prussia a powerful player in European diplomacy.

Europe's wars often spilled over to colonial outposts. American wars were therefore commonly extensions of European wars. King George's War was merely the American extension of the War of the Austrian Succession and the French and Indian War was the American extension of the larger Seven Years War (1756–1763). But in the Americas, armies had to adapt to the nature of fighting in the New World. Lacking effective roads, large urban centers, or centers of military gravity on the European model (Québec was an important exception), North American warfare often followed less formal lines. European logistics and supply systems simply could not work in the American wilderness.

Skirmishing and irregular warfare therefore became more common in America than in Europe, especially as the British and French both strove to enlist Native American nations in their wars. Ambushes and other informal tactics often proved successful in the Americas as British General Edward Braddock discovered to his dismay in 1755. Braddock tried to lead a European-style infantry column, complete with visible redcoats, fifes, and drums, through the Pennsylvania wilderness. A combined French and Indian ambush routed his men near the present-day site of Pittsburgh. Upon Braddock's death in the ambush, a young officer named George Washington helped to lead the survivors back to safety.

This process of military syncretism existed as well in India. Europeans brought their military technology and systems of training to India as a part of their processes of colonial expansion. Both England and France instilled European-style discipline into Indian armies and integrated Indian troops, called sepoys, into their systems. Sepoys were normally trained and commanded by European officers and often wore European-style uniforms. Many of these uniforms were more suited to service in Scotland or Normandy than in the hot Indian subcontinent.

During the period under study here, the military power of European states increased dramatically, often at the expense of non-European states. To explain this "rise of the west," one must look both at the integration of gunpowder weapons into European militaries and at the political, economic, and cultural changes in Europe as well. Europeans did not invent gunpowder, nor were they the first civilization to realize its military potential. Europe was, however, the first civilization to have the precise environment within which gunpowder weapons could proliferate.

Legacies

Two obvious legacies from this period stand out. First, access to guns and the administration and training needed to effectively use them proved to be dominant on battlefields across the world. Europe's ability to take the early lead in gunpowder warfare produced both an increase in warfare on the continent itself (as well as in colonies controlled by European states) and one of the key resources needed for imperialism to develop. Across the Americas and Asia, especially, Europeans, despite their numerical inferiority, carved out new empires and used their guns to control vast areas against the will of native peoples.

The second, related, legacy involves the centralization of state power that guns facilitated. Centralized governments grew markedly stronger in this period in large measure thanks to their near-monopoly of gunpowder weapons. New financial and logistical administrations created the features of the modern European state. The need to field and maintain reliable armies served as a key motivating factor.

In the next chapter we will examine how Europeans took their gunpowder advantages a step further and extended their colonial holdings. As Braddock's defeat proved, guns alone did not guarantee victory, but the battlefield power of these weapons could not be denied. Indeed, as Braddock's opponents knew, ambushing an army before it could bring its guns to bear vastly increased the chances for success. Still, guns produced a larger difference between wealthy and poor armies than had previously existed.

The introduction of gunpowder weapons must therefore be regarded as one of the most important developments in military and world history. When combined with men trained and able to use them, they made possible the creation of modern states, the decline of feudalism, and the onset of imperialism. The next major development in the history of warfare would come with the rise of nationalism, first in North America then, even more revolutionarily, in France. Sophisticated weapons would therefore become wedded to men motivated by an entirely new set of values. The result changed the nature of warfare forever.

Further reading

Carlo Cipolla, *Guns, Sails, and Empires: Technological Innovation and the Early Phases of European Expansion, 1400–1700* (Manhattan, Kansas: Sunflower Press, 1965) provides a brief and readable introduction to European acceptance of gunpowder weapons. William McNeill, *The Pursuit of Power: Technology, Armed Force, and Society Since 1000 A.D.* (Chicago: University of Chicago Press, 1983) provides another. See also: Noel Perrin, *Giving Up the Gun: Japan's Reversion to the Sword, 1543–1879* (Boulder, Colorado: Shambhala, 1979); Geoffrey Parker, *The Military Revolution: Military Innovation and the Rise of the West, 1500–1800*, third edition (Cambridge: Cambridge University Press, 1995); Paul Kennedy, *The Rise and Fall of the Great Powers: Economic Change and Military Conflict From 1500 to 2000* (New York: Vintage Books, 1989); Geoffrey Parker, ed., *The Thirty Years War* (London: Routledge, 1997).

Chapter 4

Nationalism and industrialism

Tsushima Straits, 1905

When war broke out between Russia and Japan in 1904, most Europeans expected the much larger Russian military to win easily. Just two generations earlier, Japan had been in a self-imposed isolation from westerners, unaware of the many recent changes in warfare and inexperienced in the uses of modern military technology. Japan had routed China in the Sino-Japanese War (1894–1895), but few Europeans took victory over pre-modern and divided China as a true test of military power. Europeans had not lost a major engagement to an East Asian force since the period of imperialism had begun. Few whites expected the Russo-Japanese War to be any different.

In retrospect, however, the weaknesses of the Russian military become apparent. Russia's navy was primarily based in the Baltic Sea, facing Germany, when war broke out with Japan. Furthermore, the only year-round ice-free Russian Pacific base at Port Arthur in Manchuria was under siege by Japanese land and naval forces. The Baltic Fleet therefore had to sail halfway around the world to engage the Japanese and relieve the siege.

Although most Europeans discounted the Japanese navy, it was in fact a better force than its Russian foe. Since its "opening" to the west in 1853, Japan had quickly built a modern military based on European models. The presumably stronger Russian navy encompassed eight battleships, eight cruisers, and nine destroyers of uneven quality. Many of them were obsolete. The Japanese fleet included four battleships, eight cruisers, and twenty-one destroyers, but they were all faster and more modern than their Russian counterparts.

The Russians also faced a severe morale problem based in a domestic crisis that culminated in the Revolution of 1905. With problems at home, few Russian sailors cared for war against Japan. For the Japanese, on the other hand, a victory would mean immediate recognition and respect for their newly emergent nation and, more practically, supremacy in the Far East. Japanese sailors were, therefore, better trained, better led, and better disciplined.

Japanese Admiral Togo Heihachiro waited for the Russians in the Tsushima Straits between Japan and Korea. Togo used the superior speed of his vessels to perform the textbook naval maneuver of crossing the "T." Japan's ships, the top of the "T," cut off the Russians, who were arriving in line, forming the bottom of the "T." The Russians therefore sailed right into the full fury of superior Japanese gunnery. In one afternoon the Russians lost all of their vessels through sinking or capture. The Russians also lost 10,000 sailors. The Japanese did not lose any major vessels, just three torpedo boats. Tsushima was one of the most lopsided battles in history. On land, Japanese troops proved to be just as powerful. The siege of Port Arthur, which the Russians defended with machine guns and artillery, cost more lives than had any single piece of territory in history up to that point. Nevertheless, superior Japanese skill and morale eventually won the position and the war. The myth of white supremacy was dealt a shattering blow as Japan leapt to the status of world power.

Japan's victory was due to three factors that characterized armed forces in general in this period. First, as was true for most successful armies of this period, the Japanese armies were staffed by highly motivated men, driven largely by patriotism and service to their nation. Second, the Japanese had excellent officers, trained and educated under a modern system of professional development. Finally, they possessed superior military technology produced by an economy that had undergone a process of industrialization. Military systems that combined these three innovations dominated the age.

The men

The major themes of this period are nicely described by three fundamental "revolutions" in the military profession in the nineteenth century, as developed by historian Walter Millis. First, an ideological revolution nationalized armies and changed the motivation for why men fought. Second, a managerial revolution, represented by the general staff system, provided rational and effective leadership of men and weapons. Finally, a technological revolution introduced a new scale of killing power for the average soldier.

The ideological revolution occurred at the end of the eighteenth century with the great rise of nationalism across Europe and the Americas. This important change had long-lasting and fundamental consequences for the history of warfare. Most significantly, nationalism reoriented the basis for loyalty among the men who joined armies. Instead of fighting for money or to escape problems at home, many fought mainly for patriotism. As a result, nationalized armies, like the Japanese in 1905, fought with a spirit not seen since the early days of the Roman Republic.

The War for American Independence (1775–1781) presaged many of these changes. The war was both a civil war and a war to sever American ties to Britain. An approximately equal number of Americans were rebels (that is, in favor of independence from Great Britain), Tories (opposed to independence), and neutral. One should not, therefore, derive the image that all Americans were equally fervent in their nationalism; they were not. Moreover, many saw their primary loyalty as belonging to states or regions rather than to the more amorphous new nation being created.

Still, the American militiaman could, when he wished to do so, appear quickly, fight hard, and remain committed to fighting. He did so out of a connection to Enlightenment ideals of self-government and military service for the purpose of individual and communal betterment. Despite significant differences between colonies, they nevertheless managed to come together in the face of a common enemy and create a professional standing army for the duration of the war. The colonists still needed significant help from third parties (mostly from France, which was eager to avenge its defeat to Britain in the Seven Years War), but patriotism gave the Americans the will to continue the fight until Britain gave in.

The French Revolution marked an even more fundamental change in the nature of armies. The logic of the Revolution implied that all Frenchmen (and women) owed service to their nation. Many revolutionaries believed that a Republican army, composed of citizen-soldiers, could serve as an important check on tyranny and absolutism. The French Republic issued the *Levée en Masse* in 1793 to unite all of its people around common national goals. It was not a draft in the modern sense of the term, but it set an important national standard by decreeing that *all* citizens of France, male, female, young, and old, owed military service in some fashion. It read:

> From this moment until that in which our enemies shall have been driven from the territory of the Republic, all Frenchmen are permanently requisitioned for service in the armies. Young men will go into battle. Married men will forge arms and transport supplies. Women will make tents, uniforms, and serve in hospitals. Children will pick up rags. Old men will have themselves carried into public squares, to inspire the courage of warriors, and to preach hatred of kings and the unity of the Republic.

Frenchmen responded to the *Levée en Masse* by producing fourteen new French armies in just a few weeks.

France's Jourdan Law (1798), Europe's first large-scale systematic draft, went even further by requiring all young men in France to register for military service. By 1815 the Jourdan system had provided 2,000,000 men to the Revolutionary and Napoleonic armies. Soon other states in Europe were trying to imitate both the national spirit of the *Levée en Masse* and the quantitative success of the Jourdan system.

Napoleon Bonaparte entered the scene at the perfect time to take advantage of all of the energies unleashed by nationalism. He did more to change warfare than any other individual in this period. His armies, motivated by loyalty both to him personally and to the nation of France (which many men, Napoleon above all, saw as the same entity), marched further, suffered more, and fought harder than any other. This new martial and national spirit in the hands of a man of such singular military genius produced a French empire that undermined the *ancien régime* from Spain to Russia and restructured the nature and purpose of armies.

Despite efforts by conservatives to stem the tide of the changes that Napoleon introduced, European militaries would never be the same. Armies came increasingly to serve as important national, rather than royal or dynastic, symbols. Republicans in Europe often viewed mandatory military service as a means to nationalize young men. Armies should train men to fight, republicans argued, but they could at the same time inculcate pride in national traditions, teach the national language to peasants who still spoke local dialects, and create an important personal link between men and their nation. This approach changed the average European's view of his nation's military from an instrument of oppression into an institution that, while at times still unpleasant, served necessary national goals.

Nationalism also implied changes in the relationship between aristocrats and commoners. In effect, national loyalty and patriotism became more important than aristocratic birth. Noble holds on the officer corps weakened as armies grew larger in the nineteenth century, partly as a result of Napoleon's efforts to open his military to talent rather than to birth. By 1805, half of his officers had been promoted from the enlisted ranks. In some nations, such as Prussia (after 1871 Prussia became Germany), conservative officers argued against expanding armies too much on the grounds that doing so would require allowing too many non-nobles to become officers. Nevertheless, as the military increasingly came to need skills that mirrored the skills of civilian society, nobles (who ordinarily lacked such skills) became less central in certain areas. The financial, administrative, and logistical corps of armies therefore came to be dominated by the middle class.

The increasing incorporation of civilian skills into the military also led to a greater sophistication of the military as a profession. Population increase in Europe (from 187,000,000 in 1800 to 401,000,000 in 1900) created a need to educate and train better military leaders to manage ever larger armies. Armies, especially their officer corps, therefore became more professional. In the first half of the nineteenth century military academies opened in France, Prussia, Bavaria, Russia, England, and the United States. Naval academies opened in England, France, and the United States. European armies also abolished commission by purchase and introduced promotion by merit and competitive exam rather than by noble rank or seniority.

Prussia took the lead between 1806 and 1814 with a series of reforms in response to humiliations suffered at the hands of Napoleon. The Prussians created a war academy to train middle-grade officers in the necessary theoretical and practical matters of warfare. The Prussians also created the modern general staff system in the same time period. Taking a cue from the Napoleonic staff system, the Prussian system consisted of technician-officers who advised field commanders. The Prussians extended the system to include fields like intelligence collection and analysis, contingency planning, and doctrinal development. This system created what historian Dennis Showalter has called a "nervous system" for militaries. Above all, it allowed for deeper and more complex war planning and preparation.

The success of the general staff system contributed significantly to Prussia's three quick and decisive victories in the middle of the nineteenth century. The Prussians easily defeated Denmark in 1864, beat Austria in just seven weeks in 1866, and then humbled France in 1870–1871. After these wars, the benefits of a general staff seemed manifest to contemporaries. The Prussian/German general staff grew from eighty-eight officers in 1867 to 650 by 1914. Most modern militaries endeavored to create a general staff of their own, although not all general staffs followed the Prussian model. Austria created its own staff within seven years of losing the Seven Weeks War. France followed suit in 1883 (also largely in response to the loss to Prussia); the United States created a staff in 1903; Britain and Russia did so in 1906.

Ideas about nationalism spread across the globe, fueling military activities as a natural consequence. Nationalism nearly led the independence-minded Boers of South Africa to a victory over the much wealthier British Empire during the Boer War (1899–1902). But not all emerging nations could easily translate national vigor into military power. In some places, like the United States during the Civil War (1861–1865), competing visions of nationalism led to brutal and violent internal wars. In other areas, imperialists fought long and hard to suppress national sentiment among subjugated peoples. Once again, near-constant warfare in Europe forced reforms that, generally speaking, made European militaries stronger than non-European militaries.

The machines

This period represents an age of increasing refinement in weapons technologies and new innovations in auxiliary technologies, most significantly in the fields of transportation and communication. The industrial revolution greatly enhanced the production of weapons both by increasing the sheer volume of arms produced and by increasing the quality of those arms. The ability of industrialized nations to convert their economic power into military prowess quickly provided significant battlefield advantages. More industrialized societies held important advantages over less industrial ones, as witnessed most obviously in the American Civil War, the Spanish-American War (1898), the Sino-Japanese War, and the Russo-Japanese War.

Even before the full onset of industrialization, the so-called "American system of mass production" improved arms production through the principles of standardization and interchangeability. All parts produced under this system were manufactured to exact, identical specifications. Such parts were therefore easier to stock and keep close at hand. These innovations simplified manufacturing, maintenance, and repair. Industrialization allowed such parts and finished goods to be made in quantity.

Industry and the principles of manufacturing made possible the mass production of weapons formerly limited by the craft and skill of a small number of experts. Rifling was one such technology. A rifle differs from a musket because the former has a groove cut into the inside of its barrel. When the bullet or cartridge is fired, it naturally heats and expands into the groove. It then spirals as it leaves the gun, vastly increasing both its range and accuracy; think of the difference between an American football thrown by grasping the laces as opposed to one thrown by pushing it from one end. Whereas an individual musket could rarely hit the proverbial broadside of a barn at 100 yards, a rifle could effectively strike a target the size of a man from as far away as 300 yards. In the hands of an expert sharpshooter, its effective range could be as long as 1,000 yards. Recall that Wolfe had to let the French troops at Québec in 1759 get as close as forty yards from his line before his own troops could accurately fire. In 1863 at the Battle of Gettysburg, by contrast, rifled small arms and artillery withered Confederate troops from distances as great as half a mile. The result was the death of more than half of the men who attempted "Pickett's Charge."

The concept of rifling was not new. The Chinese had understood the principle for centuries and the American rebels used a limited number of rifles with deadly effectiveness against the British in the War for American Independence. By the 1840s, however, mass production techniques made standardized rifles easier and cheaper to manufacture. By the time of the Crimean War (1854–1856) rifles were standard issue, as were mass-produced bullets called "minié balls" that were hollowed out at the bottom to facilitate the expansion of lead flanges i . the rifle's grooves.

Over time, small arms improved even further. Breech-loading rifles, standard issue in Prussia by 1851, enabled men to fire and reload while lying down. Metallic cartridges further .. ved the efficiency of rifles by limiting the amount of propellant gases that escaped. Breech-loading and metallic cartridges also increased the rate of fire seven-fold over muzzle-loaders. Finally, smokeless powder allowed the shooter to fire without giving away his position. The key point is that over the course of the period under study in this chapter, the average soldier's individual killing power increased dramatically.

As in small arms, rifling and other innovations also dramatically improved the lethality of heavy guns. A smoothbore cannon of the type used by Napoleon had an effective range of 1,000 yards and could fire two rounds per minute. By the 1870s, breech-loaded and rifled artillery could fire ten rounds per minute as far as three miles. Over the course of the nineteenth century, science and industry provided stronger propellants and developed mechanisms to reduce recoil, further increasing the utility of artillery. Although most commanders were slow to realize it, the tactical advantage had swung to the defense. The massed charges that Napoleon used with such great effectiveness in the first decade of the nineteenth century became suicidal by the middle of the century.

Near the end of the American Civil War, rapid-fire weapons appeared. The first effective types, called Gatling guns, were hand-cranked and jammed frequently. The Americans, who lacked an entrenched military class to oppose military innovation and an entrenched class of skilled arms craftsmen to oppose industrialization, became the center of innovation and production for rapid-fire weapons. Around 1884, American inventor Hiram Maxim developed what is now considered the first true "automatic gun" which used the force of recoil to eject the spent cartridge, then load and fire the next one. He was soon demonstrating his gun to military and political leaders across the United States and Europe.

The armies of Europe were slow to integrate automatic guns (the rhetorical linkage of "machine" and "gun" dates to World War I) into their continental forces. Many military leaders feared that such guns would destroy the traditional place of the soldier and horse on the battlefields of Europe. Furthermore, many automatic guns at this time were slow-moving and cumbersome. They did not fit neatly into the fashionable offensive military doctrines of the day. Such weapons also had to be kept as secret as possible. In the French army, the main automatic gun, the hand-cranked Montigny Mitrailleuse, was so secret that when war broke out with Prussia in 1870 hardly any French soldiers knew how to use it.

Europeans did, however, see the immense killing power of the automatic gun as a useful asset in advancing imperialism. Automatic guns allowed relatively small European armies to defeat much larger African and Asian ones. Superior weapons, automatic guns above all, made possible the relatively inexpensive control of large territories in the face of hostile native populations. In the Sudan in 1898 the British used superior weapons, including several automatic guns, to kill 11,000 Dervish troops with a loss of less than fifty of their own men. Racism blinded Europeans into thinking that superior white civilization, not automatic guns, created such lopsided victories. Thus, despite evidence in Africa and from wars like the Russo-Japanese War where automatic guns proved deadly, most Europeans missed the key lesson of the new weapons technologies.

Sea warfare changed radically as well. In the course of the time period under study in this chapter, steel replaced wood as the primary material of construction, steam replaced sail as the primary means of propulsion, and recoilless rifled artillery replaced smoothbore cannon as the main armament. As they proved at Tsushima, Japan excelled in the application of these new technologies. Great Britain continued its dominance at sea, introducing many of the new changes and placing their rivals at a severe disadvantage. By the 1890s, British capital ships were protected by an expensive nickel-steel armor system that provided increased protection without adding weight. At the end of this period, German efforts to close the naval gap with Britain produced many of the tensions that underlay the crisis that led to World War I.

Ancillary technologies also played important roles in changing the nature of the battlefield. Railroads and the steam engine caused the first major military transportation changes in centuries. Once again, militaries that could take advantage of these changes could translate these advantages into battlefield superiority. During the American Civil War, the North's 22,000 miles of standardized (i.e., the width between the rails was all the same) railroad tracks proved to be a tremendous logistical advantage over the South's 9,000 miles of non-standardized tracks. During the course of the war, the North's industrial capacity continued to produce more railroad mileage while Northern armies made Southern railroads and railroad junctions primary targets.

Europeans also made effective use of railroads. Although primarily a civilian development, some nations soon saw the railroad's military utility. Prussia increased its rail network from just 291 miles in 1840 to 3,500 miles in 1860. Prussia's efficient use of these expanding rail communications during the Wars of German Unification (1864–1871) allowed them to quickly transfer men and supplies. Railroads were also crucial to imperialism. By 1900 Great Britain had constructed 20,000 miles of railroads in India. These lines provided the British army with an important logistical advantage in both frontier warfare and internal security operations. As locomotives changed land transportation, steam engines changed naval transportation, allowing ships to challenge previously difficult to navigate rivers, especially in Africa. Steam engines also allowed ships to move faster and take on choppier waters in the open seas. Britain and France used steam ships to provide logistical support for their troops in Russia during the Crimean War.

Communications technologies also witnessed a tremendous change. Electric telegraphs represented a watershed improvement in military communications. Telegraphy was the first communications technology to significantly improve on the flags and lights that had served armies for centuries. On the battlefield, the telegraph allowed commanders to keep in touch with several subordinates at once. It also permitted civilians to keep tabs on military leaders. During the Crimean War, government officials in London and Paris used telegraphy to stay in constant touch with their generals, much to the latter's annoyance. Radio and telephones were introduced late in this period, the former being immediately monopolized by many of the world's armies and navies as its military value was quickly realized.

The battles

The national energies unleashed by the French Revolution produced a new type of warfare, one that stunned contemporaries accustomed to the limited warfare of the eighteenth century. The Revolutionary armies, though not always the most talented or best disciplined, used their patriotic furor to defeat larger forces. One of the Revolution's most important victories came at Valmy in 1792. Prussian forces under the command of the highly respected Duke of

Brunswick approached France's frontier with Belgium with the intention of crushing the Revolution and its threat to the *ancien régime* system. Instead, rallied to cries of "Vive la nation!," French soldiers held their ground and forced Brunswick's experienced Prussians to yield. Brunswick chose not to engage the French armies and gave up his designs to advance on Paris. The Revolution was safe.

At about the same time, Napoleon was making a name for himself through charisma and brilliant command of French artillery. By 1796 he was, at age twenty-six, in command of French armies in Italy. His dramatic successes there set him upon the road to greatness. A victory in 1800 at Marengo compelled Austria and Britain to make peace, ending the War of the Second Coalition on terms favorable to France. Within four years, Napoleon was Emperor of France and Europe was again on the brink of war.

Of all of Napoleon's talents, his most important was a tenacity that shook European militaries trained to fight for limited goals. At Austerlitz in December, 1805, Napoleon defeated a larger Russian and Austrian force through operational speed and genius. He divided his forces, which were outnumbered 85,000 men to 73,000 men, in two. One half served as an anvil, while the other half hammered into the Russo-Austrian flank. The French attack, timed to occur just as the Austrians and Russians were overextending themselves, destroyed the center of the Russo-Austrian line. As his defeated enemy retreated across a frozen lake, Napoleon ordered his artillery to fire on the ice, causing Austrian soldiers to drown in the freezing water and trapping many more between French forces and the lake. Austerlitz is still considered Napoleon's masterpiece. Despite being outnumbered, he inflicted 26,000 casualties while taking less than 9,000. Time and time again, Napoleon used French élan, operational brilliance, and a commitment to total war to humble opposing forces.

But his very success laid the seeds for his defeat. His opponents, the Prussians above all, eventually learned to copy parts of his organizational system. Napoleon himself seemed not to know when to stop. His invasion of Russia in 1812 led to the French capture of Moscow, but the ensuing Russian winter destroyed his formidable *Grande Armée*. Napoleon's wars killed one in five Frenchmen born between 1790 and 1795 (this ratio astonishingly parallels that of World War I, which killed one in four Frenchmen born between 1891 and 1895). The French, moreover, never found a suitable way to deal with English sea power, nor, ironically, with the national and regional energies that invading French forces inspired in places like Spain. Despite his final defeat in 1815, Napoleon's accomplishments inspired generals for a century to try to distill and imitate the genius of the man most considered the finest general ever. Many would try to become the next Napoleon. None succeeded.

American professional soldiers after Napoleon studied the works of Baron Antoine Henri de Jomini, a Swiss military theorist who had served under Napoleon in several important campaigns. Jomini explained Napoleon's success by arguing that there were a finite number of immutable, scientific principles that guided warfare. Napoleon, he argued, had mastered the most important of these principles: massing force against a decisive point in the enemy lines. Jomini became required reading at West Point in the years leading up to the American Civil War.

Between the time of Jomini's writings and the American Civil War, however, rifles had replaced muskets. As a result, frontal charges by massed formations faced a much more lethal environment. The increased range and accuracy of rifles doomed such charges to failure. At Fredericksburg in 1862 the Union attempted fourteen separate charges at heavily defended Confederate positions, causing 12,500 Union casualties while inflicting less than 6,000 enemy casualties. The South's famous "Pickett's Charge" at Gettysburg the following year yielded similar results. Northern troops shouted "Fredericksburg" in revenge at the Southerners after their charge fell apart.

By the end of the American Civil War, exponentially increased firepower had led to the creation of a series of earthworks and trenches that foreshadowed World War I. In 1864 at the Battle of Cold Harbor, Union General Ulysses Grant attacked powerful enemy fortifications and lost 7,000 men in one hour. Confederate defenses around Petersburg, Virginia, kept that city in Confederate hands through 1864 and into April, 1865 despite repeated Union attacks and a Union detonation of a mine packed with four tons of gunpowder under the Southern lines.

The nature of the war grew increasingly harsh, especially in comparison with the gentlemanly environment of 1861. In the early days, some generals (the South's legendary Thomas "Stonewall" Jackson among them) even proposed banning combat on Sundays. By 1864, by contrast, civilians had become a routine target of military operations. Union General William Sherman's famous "March to the Sea" through Georgia and South Carolina in 1864 cut a fifty-mile wide avenue of devastation. Sherman's intent, he declared, was to make Georgia howl. His men moved on to South Carolina, the state that began secession, and burned its capital, Columbia.

Most Europeans failed to learn the crucial lessons of the American Civil War. They preferred to focus instead on Prussia's three quick victories that occurred in the same time period. These wars seemed to confirm what most Europeans wanted to believe: that fast, relatively inexpensive victories were still possible. This belief blinded Europeans to the real power of contemporary weapons. As a result, European military doctrine between 1871 and 1914 focused on offensives and the quest for a fast, decisive campaign.

In the wake of Napoleon, most Europeans sought ways to reduce war and its attendant effects on civilians. Continental conferences, treaties, and declarations formalized "rules of warfare." Blockades and sea warfare became codified and legalized in the 1856 Declaration of Paris. The Geneva Convention of 1864 protected the rights of non-combatants and medical staff. The 1907 Hague Conference tried to establish an international panel to peacefully resolve

European disputes. Non-governmental organizations dedicated to reducing the suffering of war emerged as well, the most famous example being the Red Cross in 1862.

Outside Europe, the new organizational systems and technologies gave Europeans tremendous advantages over non-Europeans, except in cases like Tsushima. Furthermore, Europeans rarely applied the same ethical or legal standards to imperial warfare that they applied to wars on the continent. In the First Opium War (1839–1842) Great Britain used its superior navy to force trade concessions on the Chinese, including the right to sell opium. With a token force of 10,000 men and just sixteen warships, England defeated the once-powerful Chinese. They were able to do so because Chinese military technology was more reminiscent of the eighteenth century than the nineteenth. One British sloop sunk fifty-eight Chinese junks without taking a single hit. As a result of the war, England gained trade ports including Hong Kong, the right of extraterritoriality, and favorable economic arrangements. The Opium War left the Chinese humbled and enfeebled.

But China's worries were not over yet. Its war against Japan (the Sino-Japanese War, 1894–1895) proves the general point about the superiority of the western system. Japan, which had reformed its military along western models, defeated China, which in the aftermath of the Opium Wars and the bloody Taiping Rebellion had not done so. The Japanese fleet looked very similar in broad outline to the British or French, with steel battleships and modern armaments. The Chinese navy still relied on antiquated wooden ships and smoothbore guns. Chinese land forces, though significantly larger than their Japanese opponents, were disorganized and unprepared for modern war. The Japanese, on the other hand, had reformed their army on the Prussian model, complete with a general staff and national conscription.

As the Russo-Japanese example clearly demonstrates, one should not confuse European superiority with European invincibility. Military advantages did not make imperialism inevitable, nor did it mean that Europeans always emerged victorious. One powerful African nation, the Zulus, put up a strong resistance to European settlement in southern Africa from the 1830s until the early twentieth century. At Isandhlwana in 1879, a Zulu force of 10,000 destroyed a column of 1,800 British soldiers and 1,000 African allies; only fifty-five British (one of whom went on to command II Corps of the British Expeditionary Force in World War I) and 300 Africans survived. Isandhlwana proves the general point of European technological superiority; one of the chief causes of the British defeat was that they ran out of bullets. A Zulu warrior's description of the event shows the courage of the Africans in the face of European military technology.

> By that time, the inGobamakhosi had got in among the [British] rockets and killed the horses, and we were circling round so as to shut in the camp on the side of the river, but we could not advance because the fire from the

donga [dry watercourse] was too heavy. The great indunas [chiefs] were on the hill to the north of the camp, and just below them a number of soldiers were engaging the umCijo regiment, which was being driven back, but one of the chiefs of the umCijo ran down from the hill and rallied them, calling out that they would get the whole impi [force] beaten and must come on. Then they all shouted "Usutu!" and waving their shields charged the soldiers with great fury. The chief was shot through the forehead and dropped down dead, but the umCijo rushed over his body and fell upon the soldiers, stabbing them with their assegais and driving them right in among the tents.[1]

A Zulu attack on a well-equipped British military hospital during the same campaign did not fare as well. Less than seventy-five able-bodied British troops used modern rifles and artillery to hold off 5,000 Zulus. The British gave eleven men their highest military honor, the Victoria Cross, for the defense of the hospital. It was then the most Victoria Crosses ever awarded for a single action.

European settlers in southern Africa, known as Boers, put up a stiff resistance against the British as well. Loosely organized into a local militia, the Boers (mostly of Dutch ancestry) used modern weapons to compensate for a general lack of knowledge of modern strategy and operations. Using repeating rifles and smokeless powder, Boer irregulars wreaked havoc on formal British units. Eventually Britain had to send 500,000 men to South Africa to subdue a Boer force that never had more than 40,000 men in the field at any one time. Britain also resorted to burning homes and farms and sending entire Boer families to relocation camps. Eventually, Britain won, but its behavior brought near-universal scorn and criticism from the international community. The Boer War foreshadowed many of the anti-colonial wars of the post-World War II period in that it pitted a larger, more technologically sophisticated force against a smaller, more determined one. In this case the former won, but the tables would turn in the post-war period (see Chapter 7).

Legacies

No previous 150 year period had witnessed such rapid change in the nature of military technologies and organizations as the one under study here. The great tragedy is that few people fully understood these changes. European generals did not systematically learn the lessons of the trench warfare that characterized the Russo-Japanese War and the American Civil War. Instead they studied the decisive victories of Napoleon and planned to win as the great general had done if called upon to do so.

Millis's analysis of the three military revolutions of this period, discussed at the beginning of this chapter, helps to explain why the next war we will examine, World War I, was so much more brutal and deadly than were the wars of the nineteenth century. These three revolutions provided armies with more motivated soldiers, more deadly weapons, and more centralized organization. Armies therefore developed tremendous staying power and were supported by the power of industrialization. Although few Europeans realized it at the time, armies had become, in the words of Dennis Showalter, doomsday machines.

Note

1 Quoted in John Keegan, *The Book of War* (New York: Viking, 1999), p. 233.

Further reading

On technological change in this period see John Ellis, *The Social History of the Machine Gun* (Baltimore: Johns Hopkins University Press, 1975); Dennis Showalter, *Railroads and Rifles: Soldiers, Technology, and the Unification of Germany* (Hamden, Conn.: Archon Books, 1975); and Walter Millis, *Arms and the State: Civil-Military Elements in National Policy* (New York: Twentieth Century Fund, 1958). Two of the most often cited contemporary works are Carl von Clausewitz, *On War* (London: Penguin, 1988) originally published in 1832, and Antoine-Henri Jomini, *The Art of War* (Novato, Calif.: Presidio, 1992), originally published in 1838. On individual wars, David Chandler, *The Campaigns of Napoleon* (New York: Macmillan, 1966) remains the standard work. See also the section on the Battle of Waterloo (1815) in John Keegan, *The Face of Battle* (New York: Penguin, 1976). Russell Weigley, *A Great Civil War: A Military and Political History* (Bloomington: Indiana University Press, 2000) is a recent treatment of the American Civil War.

Chapter 5

World War I

Gallipoli, 1915

For almost a year, British, French, and Belgian forces had opposed German forces along a system of trenches that became known as "the western front." The incredible firepower that the armies commanded produced a stalemate that neither side could break. The battles of 1914 had severely depleted Britain's highly-trained, but relatively small, professional army. The powerful Royal Navy was useless in the trenches. Several senior British officials, including the First Lord of the Admiralty, Winston Churchill, believed that the answer must come from someplace other than France. The "easterners," as they came to be known, sought a place where they could use the Royal Navy to inflict an important defeat on the Central Powers of Germany, Austria-Hungary, and Turkey.

That place turned out to be the Gallipoli Peninsula in Turkey. The British planned to use their prized battleships to force their way into the Dardanelles Straits and pressure the Turkish capital, Constantinople. They hoped to knock Turkey out of the war and open up warm-water sea communications with their struggling Russian allies. When Turkish mines and guns prevented the British ships from completing their mission, the British chose to land a force that included thousands of Australians and New Zealanders (called Anzacs) at the Gallipoli beachheads and pressure the Turkish forces from both land and sea.

In August the Allies attacked the Sari Bair Hills in hopes of finally breaking the impasse. Most Turkish officers (and their German advisers) expected the attack to come further north. One did not. Lt. Colonel Mustafa Kemal, commander of the Ottoman Nineteenth Infantry Division, correctly predicted that Allied attacks in other sectors were a diversion for a main attack on Sari Bair.

By the time Kemal arrived at the critical point of the battle his men, out of ammunition, were retreating. Kemal ordered them to hold fast, fix bayonets, and charge. When one of his men protested that they lacked the strength to attack, Kemal, understanding the extreme gravity of the situation, replied, "I do not order you to attack. I order you to die." His men obeyed, suffering tremendous losses, but keeping the Sari Bair Hills in Turkish hands long enough for reinforcements to arrive. The Gallipoli campaign remained a stalemate until the British finally evacuated the following January. The war would have to be won, or lost, on the western front.

His actions at Sari Bair made Kemal a hero. After the war he became the first president of the modern nation-state of Turkey. In London, the Gallipoli disaster (the Allies lost over 150,000 men) cost Winston Churchill, then just forty-one years old, his place in the British government. He left London and volunteered for a battalion command in the very trenches of the western front that he had hoped to eliminate.

Gallipoli is not the bloodiest or the most important campaign of World War I, but it reveals the immense global nature of the war and strategic thinking. Great Britain, already using Canadian and Indian troops in France, used Australian troops to try to knock Turkey out of the war in order to help their Russian ally. Although the bulk of the fighting in World War I occurred in Europe, the war directly touched every inhabited continent except South America, though minor naval battles were fought even there, marking the international impact of what was then known simply as The Great War.

The men

The men who fought in World War I were mostly products of large-scale military conscription and training programs that emerged in the nineteenth century. Among the major European powers, only Great Britain avoided a draft, preferring instead to invest its defense money in the Royal Navy. Conscription became a regular fact of life for hundreds of thousands of European men, creating large armies in all the major powers.

The capital cities of Europe filled in the summer of 1914 with eager young men, draftees and volunteers alike, ready to go to war. War, as it had for generations, became a test of manhood, of patriotism, and of individual honor. For some, these appeals blended with the age-old allure of warfare to provide adventure. The new soldiers were led by officers who believed that the war would be short. All sides counted on the moral and spiritual superiority of their nation's value system to produce a quick victory. Few officers were adequately prepared to deal with the realities of a long, industrial war.

They were, however, prepared to start one. European general staffs developed complicated, highly secret, and often inflexible war plans, designed to be opened and implemented at a moment's notice. The most famous of these, the German Schlieffen Plan, tried to resolve Germany's basic strategic dilemma. Stuck between a more populous Russia to the east and a vengeful France to the west, Germany needed to avoid a two-front war. The Schlieffen Plan proposed moving eighty-seven per cent of Germany's mobilized manpower against the French, encircling Paris, and defeating France in six weeks. German troops would then entrain, move east and meet the presumably slower mobilizing

Russians. The plan also involved invading the neutral country of Belgium in order to get to Paris as quickly as possible. Great Britain, eager that Germany not control Belgium's ports on the English Channel, had threatened war if Belgium were invaded.

France's Plan XVII called for French troops to move immediately into the Alsace-Lorraine region, which Germany had seized from France in 1870. The German General Staff had counted on the French putting revenge over military prudence. They therefore placed a token force in Alsace-Lorraine to pin the French down while the bulk of German forces moved west of the French army through Belgium and proceeded toward Paris. The French were slow to realize that they were falling into a trap.

War planning necessarily depended on educated guesses and gambles. The Germans gambled that the Russians would mobilize slowly, that Britain would not declare war over Belgium, that Belgium itself would not put up a strong resistance, and that France would invade Alsace-Lorraine. Only the last proved to be correct. For their part, the French gambled that Britain would declare war, that Italy would not honor its treaty obligations to Germany by invading southern France (they did not and in 1915 joined the Allies), and that the Russians would mobilize quickly enough to threaten Germany from the east. The French guessed better than the Germans; their gambles paid off. These educated guesses may very well have saved France.

Although few people realized it in 1914, war planning and rapid mobilization schemes provided the domino effect that engulfed Europe that fateful summer. The assassination of an Austrian archduke led to a series of mobilizations and implementations of war plans. Serbia, whom the Austrians accused of masterminding the murder, mobilized its small army to meet an anticipated attack from Austria-Hungary. Austria-Hungary mobilized to punish the Serbs for stirring up anti-Austrian sentiment in the Balkans. Austro-Hungarian mobilization led to Russian mobilization, both out of sympathy for the Serbian cause and out of the knowledge that mobilizing a vast country could take time. Seeing a large war quickly developing, Germany, France, the Ottoman Empire, and England soon followed.

By late 1914, the western front had bogged down into a stalemate of opposing trench systems that stretched from the English Channel to Switzerland. On the western front alone, the men dug 25,000 miles of zig-zagged trenches, enough to circle the globe if set end-to-end. The defensive nature of World War I weapons technology meant that offensive charges against these trenches, so crucial to the pre-war doctrine of all armies, were bound to fail. Nevertheless, commanders continued to order them despite horrific losses.

Some historians blame the generals for being unimaginative and tied to outmoded forms of warfare. Generalship in World War I was generally poor. Many generals, like France's Joseph Joffre, stayed far behind the lines in luxurious châteaux, ate sumptuous lunches, took regular naps, and rarely saw a wounded soldier. Few outstanding senior officers emerged. Russia's Alexei

Brusilov, Turkey's Mustafa Kemal, and France's Ferdinand Foch are three exceptions.

No written account can accurately convey the horrors of trench life. Trenches were often filled with water, mud, lice, rats, corpses, and pieces of corpses. Each side protected their trenches with barbed wire and machine gun nests, making them virtually impenetrable to infantry attack. Some German trenches went as deep as thirty feet underground. During times of heavy fighting, regular supplies of food, drinking water, medicine, and ammunition were rare. In many instances, bodies could not even be properly buried; when they were, they were often disinterred by subsequent enemy shells.

Although the western front receives the most attention, other fronts soon developed. The bloody Gallipoli front in Turkey proved ineffective as did fronts in Africa, Greece, and a bitterly contested front in the Alps between Austria-Hungary and Italy. In the latter case almost 300,000 men died during eleven separate and inconclusive battles for control of the marginally important Isonzo River valley. A poorly planned winter campaign in the Caucasus Mountains may have resulted in as many as 30,000 Turkish soldiers dying of the cold alone.

The unprecedented pounding by artillery and the continued senseless attacks sometimes proved to be too much. Doctors began to see thousands of cases of men with no physical injuries but who nevertheless exhibited evident nervous disorders. Men developed facial ticks, became catatonic, or lost the ability to walk normally. Some officers blamed the men for a lack of courage, but many soon came to recognize the problem as a serious one. Not knowing exactly what it was or how to treat it, the men tellingly called it "shell-shock." After the war, doctors came to understand that just as human bodies (especially ones suffering from poor food, exhaustion, and lack of sleep) have limits, so too do human nerves. During the war, the best doctors could often do was to remove men from the front lines, sometimes to specialized treatment centers. Some men recovered after a period of rest and treatment. Others never did.

The enormous enthusiasm of the war's early months faded as casualties mounted and the war ground on with no evidence of an end in sight. The British, having already employed Canadians, Anzacs, and Indians and still reluctant to rely heavily on conscription, introduced a system known as "Pals Battalions." Men were permitted to enlist "with their pals" for the duration of the war. When these units saw action, as the Liverpool Pals did at the Battle of the Somme, they often suffered casualties that devastated their home communities. In one day at the Somme, the Liverpool Pals had 500 of their 2,500 men killed.

The irrelevance of the individual in the trenches led to a quest for men who could fit age-old heroic models. Pilots came closest to the ideal of the modern-day knight, with the airplane as the new charger. Of course, the reality was quite different. Aviation, especially in primitive aircraft, was every bit as dangerous as trench life. Of France's 13,000 World War I aviators, 3,500 died in combat, 2,000 died in training, and another 3,000 suffered serious accidents.

Few armies issued parachutes to their men out of fear that men might be more willing to ditch their expensive airplanes at the first sign of mechanical trouble.

All of the great imperial powers looked to tap the manpower resources of their overseas empires as well. The French employed 170,000 North African and Senegalese troops and the British used Indian troops on the western front. France also used laborers from their colonies in Indochina on the western front and troops from that region in Greece. The international diversity of the war is reflected in a cemetery in Belgium near Ypres that contains the remains of 4,500 men from Great Britain, Canada, Australia, New Zealand, South Africa, India, China, and Germany.

Each side also sought to enlist additional allies to help with the fighting. Japan fought on the Allied side, seizing German colonial bases in the Pacific Ocean. Britain enlisted Arab troops, eager to rebel against the Ottoman Empire. The Allies were eventually able to call on another source of manpower, the Americans, who entered the war in part because of the effect that German submarines had on civilians. Americans appeared in large numbers in the spring of 1918 just as the Germans were making their final gamble to win the war. Eventually almost 1,000,000 Americans served "over there" and provided the crucial margin of manpower for the Allies.

The machines

In the years before the war, industrial Europe produced a multitude of weapons, the full effects of which often escaped the otherwise careful studies of general staffs. Furthermore, European industry also developed new weapons technologies and vastly improved on older ones. All of these patterns combined to make World War I a war dominated by machines.

Artillery killed more men than any other weapon. It was a fear-inspiring weapon that killed indiscriminately, maimed bodies, and was fired from such a range that soldiers hardly ever saw the men shooting at them. Among the largest pieces was the German Big Bertha, which fired 420 mm (seventeen inch) diameter shells powerful enough to penetrate steel-reinforced concrete. The ultimate expression of artillery in World War I was the so-called "Paris Gun" developed by the Germans to terrorize the French capital. It fired a 108 kg (238 lb) shell on a trajectory that took it half-way to space before it landed as far as ninety miles away. These guns required a constant flow of men and artillery shells to be sent to the front. In 1914 the French averaged 900,000 shells fired per month. By 1916 they averaged 4,500,000 shells fired per month. In 1918 the Germans averaged 8,000,000 per month. By way of comparison the Germans averaged 20,000 shells per month during the Austro-Prussian War of 1866.

Poison gas was another horrifying weapon, all the more so because of its novelty. All armies endeavored to develop better gas masks and respirators, then they endeavored to develop gases that could pass through the improved masks, inspiring a frightful game of cat and mouse. Gas was a terrifying but unpredictable weapon, subject to weather conditions. A change in wind direction might blow the gas back on one's own troops.

Its first appearance on the battlefield in April, 1915 terrified French troops at the Battle of Ypres. The Germans used 168 tons of chlorine gas (which killed by causing over-production of fluid in the lungs) from cylinders operated by artillery. Later that year, the Germans turned to a deadlier blend of chlorine and phosgene gases. The new mixture sunk into enemy trenches, making it harder for enemy troops to avoid it. In 1917, Germany introduced mustard gas, firing more than 1,000,000 shells of it at British lines in just three weeks.

If artillery seemed overwhelming to many men, gas seemed sinister, almost human, in its ability to seep down into trenches in search of its victims. The ability of a man to get to his gas mask and apply it in time could mean the difference between life and a painful death. Heavy, uncomfortable gas masks became a regular feature of life in the trenches. A man learned to keep his mask close at hand or ran a terrible risk.

Machine guns proved to be incredibly effective in repulsing charges by large numbers of men. A single machine gun could fire as many as 500 rounds a minute (or about eight rounds every second). The .30 caliber bullets fired from a Browning machine gun could penetrate masonry walls. The guns stopped even the most courageous men literally dead in their tracks. Heroism became almost irrelevant. Historian John Ellis captured the tragedy thus, "It was as simple as this: three men and a machine gun can stop a battalion of heroes."[1] In one 1915 battle two machine guns manned by twelve Germans stopped two whole battalions (1,500 men) of British infantry.

As we saw, airplanes became the very symbol of the individualistic, courageous war that many men wanted to fight. Initially, airplanes only spotted for artillery units and observed enemy movements. The airplane was, after all, a new and untested technology. The Wright brothers' famous flight at Kitty Hawk had occurred only eleven years before the outbreak of the war. Few pilots had any experience or training in aerial combat.

Within the first few months, however, men began to carry rifles and pistols into cockpits with them. Aviation combat was extremely complicated as pilots had to shoot and fly at the same time, presenting pilots with the problem of shooting around or above the arc of the propeller. Often, aviators had to stand up when they fired and might have to climb halfway out of the cockpit in midair to reload or clear jams.

Creative pilots sought ways to remedy this situation and therefore allow them to fly sitting down, keep enemy pilots in their sights, and attain reasonable degrees of both accuracy and safety. French pilots tried to solve the problem by attaching metal deflector shields to the back of wooden propellers. This innovation protected the blades, but the deflected bullets might fly anywhere, even back at the pilot.

The Germans finally solved the problem by synchronizing the propeller with the plane's machine gun. The innovation allowed the machine gun to effectively fire through the propeller arc, permitting the pilot to fly and accurately shoot at the same time. The world's first true fighter aircraft was born. The Germans introduced the plane in 1916 at the Battle of Verdun where, to keep the device secret for as long as possible, German pilots were forbidden to fly it over French lines. Until the French and British developed their own synchronizing system, German planes gained an important upper-hand.

Air power continued to grow. At the Battle of St Mihiel in 1918 the Allies concentrated 1,481 aircraft from six nations in support of a ground offensive. The air contingent included 701 fighter planes, 366 observation aircraft, and 414 bombers. The Germans, with fewer resources to devote to aviation, had just 213 aircraft in the sector. They lost the battle. By the end of the war twin-engine German Gotha bombers were able to drop incendiary bombs on London and Paris, bringing the terror of the war to civilians. The most deadly of the raids killed 259 Parisians, a number that seems small to contemporary readers, but a terrible demonstration of a novel weapon to people in 1918.

Submarines also increased the death toll of civilians. All of the great powers had submarines, but Germany made the most effective use of them. In 1915, U-boats sank 227 British ships for a total of 855,721 gross tons. In the first half of 1916 they sank 610,000 gross tons before Germany decided to reduce activity out of fears of American response. U-boats presented Germany with a tremendous weapon, but they could not follow international rules of warfare designed for surface vessels. Unrestricted submarine warfare therefore inevitably led to deaths of non-combatants from neutral countries, notably Americans. The 1915 sinking of the *Lusitania* off the south coast of Ireland killed 1,200 people including 128 Americans. The 1916 sinking of the *Sussex* increased tensions again and led to a temporary German promise not to sink passenger vessels without warning.

The next year, Germany decided to resume unlimited submarine warfare. That decision so scared Britain's senior admiral that he warned that Britain could lose the war at sea in six months. German U-boats were soon sinking one in four ships that left British ports. The German decision also played a major role in America's decision to declare war against Germany in April, 1917.

The Allies eventually developed a convoy system that solved the U-boat menace. In a convoy, warships accompanied large groupings of merchant ships, forcing submarines to remain submerged and thus incapable of firing their torpedoes. British admirals were slow to accept convoying out of fears that the U-boats would just have a larger range of targets available to them. Faced with the new threat, however, they had no choice. Convoys became the key to stopping the losses. Within a year British shipping losses to U-boats fell from twenty-five per cent of all ships leaving port to four per cent.

Convoys relied on the large surface fleet of the Royal Navy, built around Dreadnoughts, modern battleships that outclassed every battleship that had previously existed. First introduced in 1906, Dreadnoughts combined heavy armor, twelve-inch guns, and turrets capable of all-around fire. A Dreadnought could sink a standard battleship before that battleship's guns could even get in range to fire. Dreadnoughts inspired an enormously expensive arms race across Europe that led to unprecedented naval construction bills. For all of the resources that went into them, however, they did not see much action. Only one large-scale naval battle, the inconclusive 1916 Battle of Jutland, took place.

Other technologies also made their appearance. Germany introduced modern flame-throwers in 1916. In the same year, Britain introduced the tank. At the Battle of the Somme, the British brought up forty-seven of the slow, underpowered devices. Only eleven made it into the fighting. In 1917, Britain concentrated 200 tanks at the Battle of Cambrai, but, again, mechanical problems plagued them. Primitive though they were, they made a deep impression on some of the men who saw them, including Heinz Guderian, who went on to build the famous German Panzer Corps of World War II.

The battles

Many of the battles of World War I, especially on the western front, share a tragic similarity. Despite the intentions of officers who tried to find a way around the stalemate, the same features characterized most battles, including: artillery bombardments or gas attacks to "prepare" the enemy trenches; infantry assaults designed to capture those trenches; and the failure of those attacks in the face of rapid machine-gun fire. Much of the military history of the western front in World War I can be explained by the attempts to avoid these extremely costly infantry attacks and the bloody stalemates that resulted.

The German army, ready to carry out the Schlieffen Plan, put its armies into the fields fastest and with the greatest efficiency. They were, however, counting on being able to move quickly through Belgium. Although superior German artillery successfully dispatched Belgian forts, German army commanders were surprised by the strong resistance put up by Belgian armies and citizens. Belgian resistance threatened the delicate timetable required by the Schlieffen Plan. Germany responded with *Schrecklichkeit*, or frightfulness. When the medieval city of Louvain resisted, the Germans destroyed the entire town, including its irreplaceable library, one of the most valuable in Europe. The Germans burnt villages and generally ignored the laws of warfare. The propaganda value of "poor little Belgium" to the Allies notwithstanding, there was little Britain and France could do to save it. They had other problems.

France's Plan XVII had turned into a disaster. In Alsace-Lorraine, brightly-uniformed and lightly-armed French troops attacked well-fortified German positions with tremendous losses. Over 27,000 Frenchmen died in attacks on 22 August 1914, then the bloodiest day in the history of France (a dubious distinction that it would not hold for very long). As French armies moved into Alsace-Lorraine, moreover, German armies moved through Belgium and into France. The French government followed thousands of Parisians out of the city and headed for Bordeaux. It seemed to many Frenchmen that the capital might be besieged within a matter of days.

Then, the "Miracle of the Marne" saved Paris and maybe France itself. The Germans had weakened the attacking forces of the Schlieffen Plan in order to send troops east against Russia earlier than they had planned. Just twenty-five miles away from the French capital and lacking the extra troops, General Alexander von Kluck decided not to try to encircle Paris. Instead, he swung his army to the east of the city, toward the Marne River. In one of the first effective uses of military aviation, French pilots detected the German movement. This vital intelligence told French commanders that Paris would not be encircled from the north and west. It also meant that a German flank would be exposed. If French forces acted quickly, they might be able to stop the German army and the Schlieffen Plan in its tracks.

To do so, they would need to move troops out of Paris and up to the Marne River. The military commander of Paris was an innovative sixty-five year-old general named Joseph Simon Galliéni who came out of retirement when the war broke out. Galliéni organized French troops inside Paris and dispatched them to the Marne with great efficiency, giving General Joseph Joffre the resources he needed to stop the German advance. As part of Galliéni's miracle, he rushed 6,000 recent arrivals from train stations to the front by commandeering Paris' taxicabs. French troops took heavy losses, but finally stopped the German advance.

In the east, the Germans took on the advancing Russians at the titanic clash known as the Battle of Tannenberg. A German lieutenant colonel, Max Hoffman, devised a plan to drive German forces between the two main Russian armies commanded by Aleksander Samsonov and Pavel Rennenkampf. Hoffman had been a German observer in the Russian armies during the Russo-Japanese War of 1904–1905. He allegedly knew that the two Russian commanders were bitter rivals and shared a deep personal animosity. He guessed that Rennenkampf would be reluctant to place his army in a position to support that of Samsonov.

While one division held the indecisive Rennenkampf at bay, the rest of the German Eighth Army struck a surprised Samsonov in late August. Without support, Samsonov's army suffered a crushing defeat. The Russians lost 30,000 killed and a remarkable 125,000 POW compared to the loss of less than 15,000 Germans. Samsonov committed suicide as the Germans turned on Rennenkampf, inflicting another 125,000 casualties at the Battle of the Masurian Lakes in September. Incompetent leadership thus ruined Russian plans to invade Germany.

Incompetence was not a feature unique to the Russians. Even as late as 1917, British strategy consisted of offensives that held to the basic tactic of artillery preparation and infantry charge. That fall, Sir Douglas Haig ordered an offensive in the lowlands of Flanders near the scene of the First and Second Battles of Ypres. By the fall of 1917, Haig should have known better than to believe that pre-1914 tactics could overcome 1917 weapons technology. The battle, which became known as Passchendaele, followed the same lethal pattern as most of those that preceded it. But at Passchendaele, torrential rains turned the fields of Flanders into a sea of mud, literally drowning men and animals alive. By the time Haig finally called the offensive off, the British had lost 244,000 men, 66,000 of them killed, to gain eight miles.

For the remainder of the war, generals sought ways around the problem of trench warfare. Rather than try to review all of the major campaigns, let's examine the alternatives to trench warfare that generals sought. Some proved effective; most did not.

Option #1: Develop new technology. As we have seen, airplanes, tank, and other technologies failed to provide the neat, technological solution that many had hoped for. They did, however, add important new weapons that, when intelligently used in combination with existing arms, could provide limited advantages.

Option #2: Create other fronts. By the middle of 1916 there were fronts in Russia, the Caucasus Mountains, Persia, Mesopotamia, Greece, Italy, East Africa, and the Sinai Peninsula. There were also naval fronts in the Pacific Ocean and in the North Atlantic. As we saw earlier in this chapter, the British also tried to open a front on the Gallipoli Peninsula. None of these fronts proved decisive, but all brought the effects of the war to people in areas far removed from the competition of western Europe.

In East Africa German General Paul von Lettow-Vorbeck led an African army commanded by German officers and NCOs. This army, called the *Schutztruppe*, used a blend of European and African tactics to frustrate British attempts to destroy them. With no more than 11,000 African guerrillas and porters at any one time, Lettow-Vorbeck held out until two weeks after the armistice ended the war in Europe despite Britain's larger forces and command of the seas. He was able to do so because his troops knew the terrain of East Africa and taught their German officers how to make the best use of it. The *Schutztruppe* used European weapons and African tactics such as quick hit-and-run raids on British outposts and a scorched earth policy that forced civilians to support the *Schutztruppe* or pay a heavy price. Almost 15,000 African troops died as a direct result of World War I in Africa. Lettow-Vorbeck's tactics created a famine that killed thousands more and left East Africa in a weakened state to fight off the arrival of a deadly influenza epidemic there in 1919.[2]

In the Middle East, a British officer named T. E. Lawrence (also known as Lawrence of Arabia) worked with rival Arab groups anxious to achieve independence from the Ottoman Empire. Lawrence, who spoke Arabic and had lived in the Middle East, understood that European tactics and organization would not work in the very different environment of Palestine and Arabia. He secured British supplies and a promise of British support for Arab independence after the war then worked closely with Arab leader Emir Faisal to learn Arab tactics. Together Lawrence and Faisal's force of about 6,000 men tied down 25,000 Ottoman troops, captured the Ottoman stronghold of Wejh, cut the vital Hejaz Railway, seized the Red Sea port of Aqaba, and captured the Syrian city of Damascus.

After the war, Lawrence attended the Versailles Peace Conference with Faisal to complete the independence of the Arab states. There, Lawrence learned of a conflicting promise Great Britain had made to Jewish groups pledging that Palestine would one day be a Jewish homeland. The British had also signed an agreement with France that divided former Ottoman territories in the Middle East between the two European states. Both the Arabs and the Jews left Versailles disappointed and the troubled modern period of Middle Eastern history had begun, another long shadow of World War I.

Option #3: Tactical evolution: Germany developed "storm troop" tactics that involved a brief, intense bombardment followed by the rapid advance of elite light troops that bypassed enemy strong points in favor of attacks on communications and reserve positions. With enemy artillery, reserves, supply, and communication thus eliminated, German reserves then advanced and took on the enemy's main forces. These tactics broke Russian positions at Riga in September 1917 and destroyed the Italians at Caporetto in October and November.

Such tactics formed the basis of Germany's last gamble, the Ludendorff Offensives of 1918. Ludendorff, who planned the Caporetto offensive and was now in command of German forces, realized that Germany's only chance at victory was to win on the western front in spring, 1918 before the Americans began to arrive *en masse*. His use of storm troop tactics created movement in France once again, bringing German troops within fifty miles of Paris and causing another evacuation of the French government to Bordeaux. Five separate German drives pushed the Allies back, but could not break them apart.

Option #4: Use the stalemate to your advantage. German General Erich von Falkenhayn, an extremely tough man even by German army standards, planned to use the stalemate to Germany's advantage. He decided to attack the French at a place so important that they would have no choice but to defend it to the last man. As they sent troops, Falkenhayn planned to "bleed the French army white." In other words, he planned to force the French to attack, knowing that the likely result was a battle of unprecedented carnage.

He chose Verdun, a fortified town with a history of stout resistance to Germany. First taken by Germans in 923, France took it back in 1552. In 1792, its commander chose suicide rather than hand the fort over to Germans and in 1870 it was the last French fort to surrender in the Franco-Prussian War. Falkenhayn knew that France would fight just as hard for this sacred place in

1916. From 21 February to 18 December 1916 the French and Germans fought as bitter and bloody a battle as any in human history. French commanders ordered that any ground lost be immediately retaken at any price. By the time it was over, the French had indeed bled (suffering an astounding 542,000 casualties) but so had the Germans (434,000 casualties). The lines were almost the same at the end of the battle as they had been at the start.

Option #5: Improve command structures. The near collapse of the Italians at Caporetto finally convinced the Allies to name French General Ferdinand Foch supreme commander in March, 1918 just as the Germans were launching the Ludendorff Offensives. Foch controlled a strategic reserve of men from all of the allied nations that allowed him to move troops across the western front and quickly counterattack German troops worn out from their offensives.

At a Second Battle of the Marne in July 1918 French, British, Italian, and American troops fought together, riding a tide of rising morale and pushing the Germans away from Paris. On another sector of the front, the British attacked at Amiens capturing 15,000 German POW in one day. That "black day" at Amiens led Ludendorff to conclude at last that Germany had lost. Foch's wisdom and the ability of the Allies to coordinate military activity under him provided a critical element to Allied success.

Option #6: Wait for help. This option was only open to the Allies. After America's entry into the war in April, 1917, the Allies had only to hold on until the arrival of hundreds of thousands of fresh, if inexperienced, men. American entry became even more important after the Bolshevik victory in the Russian Civil War. The new Soviet government signed an armistice with the Germans in December, 1917, allowing the Germans to transfer men and arms to the western front. American troops, arriving at the rate of 10,000 men every day, more than made up the difference.

Legacies

So much had been lost in World War I for so little gained. By most reliable estimates, the war directly killed 12,000,000 people. A further 21,000,000 soldiers were wounded; many of them required medical care for the rest of their lives. The industrial nature of the war led to four years of unprecedented killing and maiming. It instilled in traumatized generals and politicians alike the desire to avoid a repeat. Some nations, like France, Britain, and the United States, sought to do so by withdrawing into isolation. Others, like Germany and Japan, looked to technological and doctrinal solutions to ensure that the next war would not be fought in trenches.

The military legacies of World War I are two-fold. First, the pressures to win the war led to the introduction of an array of terrifying new weapons. Airplanes, tanks, submarines, flame throwers, and many others got their first real combat tests. When a total war mindset combined with these new weapons systems, the result was an unprecedented level of suffering for combatants and non-combatants alike. In the years between the two world wars these weapons continued to be refined. They would all return to kill again.

The second legacy can be summed up in the often-heard phrase "Never Again." But "Never Again" meant something different to each of the great powers. To France, it meant never again fight a bloody war that destroys your homeland. To England, it meant never again fight such a terrible war on the continent. To America, it meant never again fight a war to attempt to right a fundamentally corrupted Europe. To Germany, it meant never again be humiliated. The greatest tragedy of World War I is that millions of veterans of the war lived to see (and in some cases played a role in realizing) all of the Never Agains happen to the next generation.

The Never Agains returned because the war did not solve the bitter rivalries of Europe. If anything, it only made them worse. Rather than "make the world safe for democracy" as President Wilson had hoped, it only served to make the world an even more uncertain place. Fascism and Bolshevism rose on currents of popular discontent either caused by or aggravated by the war. In World War I's wake came a bitter and resentful Germany, searching for scapegoats to remove the sting of the harsh Treaty of Versailles which stripped Germany of all of its overseas colonies and fourteen per cent of its European territory. The treaty also dismantled the German military, forced Germany to accept war guilt, and required it to pay war reparations (as it had required France to do in 1871). Ferdinand Foch, military adviser to French Prime Minister Georges Clemenceau, saw the final peace in 1919 and declared, "This is not peace. It is an armistice for twenty years." Almost twenty years to the day, the Germans invaded Poland, sparking World War II and fulfilling Foch's eerie prophecy.

Notes

1 J. Ellis, *The Social History of the Machine Gun* (Baltimore: Johns Hopkins University, 1975), p. 123.
2 I am grateful to Michelle Moyd for sharing her paper "Our Loyal Askari: Continuities in Warfare from Maji Maji and World War I" (unpublished paper, Cornell University, 2000).

Further reading

Good general introductions include John Keegan, *The First World War* (New York: Knopf, 1998); James Stokesbury, *A Short History of World War I* (New York: William Morrow, 1981); Jay Winter and Blaine Baggett, *The Great War and the Shaping of the Twentieth Century* (New York: Penguin, 1996); and Martin Gilbert, *The First World War* (New York: Henry Holt, 1994). Other standouts include Paul Fussell, *The Great War and Modern Memory* (Oxford: Oxford University Press, 1980); Alistair Horne,

The Price of Glory: Verdun 1916 (New York: St Martin's, 1963); Douglas Porch, *March to the Marne: The French Army, 1871–1914* (Cambridge: Cambridge University Press, 1981); Jay Winter, *Sites of Memory, Sites of Mourning: The Great War in European Cultural History* (Cambridge: Cambridge University Press, 1995); Hew Strachan, ed., *World War I: A History* (Oxford: Oxford University Press, 1998) which contains essays on Africa and the Middle East; and David Trask, *The AEF and Coalition Warmaking* (Lawrence: University Press of Kansas, 1993). For Africa see Charles Miller, *Battle for the Bundu: The First World War in East Africa* (New York: Macmillan, 1974).

Chapter 6

World War II

Stalingrad (1942–1943)

In June, 1941, the German army, convinced that their Russian enemies were sub-humans and thus inferior soldiers, invaded the Soviet Union. They were confident that they could win a victory in four weeks, in part because of their presumed racial superiority and in part because of their six-week victory over France the previous spring. But despite huge territorial gains, the easy victory over the Soviets remained elusive. By August, the Germans had suffered 400,000 casualties and their logistical lines were strung out across hundreds of miles of inhospitable Russian steppe. Furthermore, German beliefs that the war would be quick left them materially unprepared for the unforgiving Russian winter. With no winter oils, German vehicles could not move and with little winter clothing, soldiers froze. During that winter, the Germans evacuated more than 100,000 soldiers due to frostbite. By June, 1942 the war in Russia was further from a successful conclusion than it had been the year before.

For the Russians, the situation looked scarcely better. They had withstood the German onslaught thus far, but just barely. Millions of Russians were now prisoners of war and the Germans had come close enough to Moscow to see the spires of the Kremlin and force the removal of Lenin's body from his tomb. By summer, 1942 the Germans sought to seize the oil fields of southern Russia. As part of the operation the German Sixth Army moved to seize the city of Stalingrad. Russian leader Joseph Stalin, who had named the city for himself, ordered the Red Army to save the city or die fighting. Any Russian, military or civilian, who tried to desert was to be shot by the Soviet secret police (as an estimated 13,500 were). A titanic battle for Stalingrad began.

The battle for Stalingrad lasted throughout the summer, fall, and winter of 1942 and into 1943. At times, the fighting devolved to street-to-street, building-to-building combat. In a few of the city's structures, the fighting was floor-to-floor and room-to-room. Both sides threw every available resource into the fight. The Soviets brought in the man who had saved Moscow the previous year, General Georgi Zhukov, one of the war's greatest military minds. Stalin called on Zhukov to save Stalingrad as he had saved Moscow.

In November, amid the first snows of the coming winter, the Russians counterattacked and, thanks to Zhukov's brilliant plan and the inability of the Germans to resupply their men, they relieved the siege of the city and encircled the German Sixth Army. In late January, 1943, cut off from the rest of the German armies, the Sixth Army surrendered its remaining 91,000 starving and freezing soldiers, including twenty-two generals. In all, the Stalingrad campaign cost the Germans 500,000 men, their confidence, and their momentum. The campaign had cost the Russians more than 1,000,000 men, but Russian morale soared. Now they would have the chance to move west and avenge the cruelty of the occupying Germans.

The battle for Stalingrad impacted civilians like no battle before it. The German Air Force killed 40,000 residents of the city in one week of bombings. Still, Stalin steadfastly refused to even consider removing civilians. Instead he ordered them into action. When the Germans captured sections of the city, they executed any Russian suspected of partisan activity. They deported 60,000 more civilians to slave labor camps; few survived. In the end, less than 10,000 civilians survived; only nine children were reunited with both of their parents. Stalingrad demonstrated the horror and brutality of a war based on racial ideology and fought to the last person – military or civilian.

The men and women

Two important differences exist between those who fought World War I and World War II. First, the totality of the war, even compared to World War I, meant that old ideas of combatant and non-combatant melted away. Although civilians have always suffered as an indirect result of warfare, during World War II civilians died by the millions as a result of direct and intentional targeting. Accurate statistics are hard to come by and the numbers themselves are so large that they lose much of their meaning, but most estimates place the civilian death toll near 28,000,000 in addition to the more than 22,000,000 military deaths. Another 30,000,000 civilians became refugees. Without belittling deaths from earlier wars, compare these numbers with World War I when the 1,200 deaths aboard the *Lusitania* in 1915 created an international crisis.

World War II was a war of ideologies. Some of these ideologies, notably that of Nazi Germany, were based in pseudo-science and a warped version of Social Darwinism that argued that life was a struggle between races. Both the Japanese and the Germans based their systems on deranged notions of racial purity and the need to subdue or destroy inferior races. Racism, which had helped to sustain European justifications for colonialism and imperialism, now became fuel for motivating men to fight on behalf of their nation and their race. The ensuing racially-motivated war (what the Germans called *Rassenkampf*) created terrible atrocities, especially when the opposing sides saw themselves as members of competing racial groups.

As a direct result, civilians became targets in ways that continue to horrify people more than a half century later. Nazi ideology in particular targeted civilians who were *Untermenchen* (sub-human). This group included Jews, 6,000,000 of whom died at German hands in the Holocaust, as well as Slavs and gypsies. During World War I, most civilian casualties were largely by-products of military operations; with the important exception of the Armenian genocide, armies rarely targeted civilians. In World War II civilian deaths were the result of carefully designed plans of extermination. At times, German units dedicated themselves to finding and killing *Untermenchen*, even when their military services were badly needed in front-line military operations. In other words, racism's need to destroy racial enemies superseded the battlefield's need for maximum effectiveness.

Historian Omer Bartov has recently argued that the German Army's dedication to *Rassenkampf* left its soldiers morally anaesthetized on the eve of their invasion of Russia in June, 1941. German commanders broke all connections with international law and morality by issuing the "Barbarossa Jurisdiction Decree," which exempted German soldiers from punishment for any crime committed against Soviet civilians. Many generals, such as Walther von Reichenau and Erich von Manstein, encouraged their troops to fight an especially vicious war against Soviet and Polish civilians (10,000,000 and 4,000,000 of whom died, respectively). Special units, known as *Einsatz-gruppen*, systematically murdered Jewish and Slavic civilians throughout the Eastern Front. Soviet responses were equally as harsh as their forces moved west. Approximately 2,000,000 German civilians died during the course of the war.

Japanese treatment of East Asia proved to be no less cruel. Approximately 7,500,000 civilians died in China alone, though some scholars argue that starvation and disease (some of it a result of fighting between Chinese Nationalists and Communists) may have raised that number to as many as 20,000,000. Japanese soldiers in December, 1937 rampaged through the city of Nanking, killing, looting, raping, and torturing. Although exact numbers continue to be debated, the death toll over two days may have reached as high as 200,000. The Japanese also forced as many as 200,000 mostly Korean "comfort women" to service the sexual needs of its soldiers.

Technology contributed to the increased blurring of the distinction between combatants and non-combatants. Though not on the same immoral plane as the Axis atrocities discussed above, strategic bombing, used most often by the Americans, British, and Germans, targeted industrial centers and, at times, population centers. Aerial bombardment, which cannot easily discriminate between military and non-military targets, killed approximately 1,500,000 civilians. The Spanish Civil War (1936–1939) gave a preview of the horrors of aerial warfare. At least eight Spanish cities were the targets of air attacks. In one famous example, the German Kondor Legion, acting on behalf of the Spanish Nationalists, destroyed the Basque town of Guernica in 1937 with heavy explosives and incendiaries. The pilots also machine-gunned the town's inhabitants, sparking an international outcry.

By the middle of World War II, aerial bombardment had become such a common occurrence that Guernica faded from memory. The industrial capacity of the combatants meant that newer, heavier bombers were always being produced. The largest included the American B-17 and B-29 bombers and the British Lancaster, each capable of carrying 20,000 pounds of bombs. All told, the Allies built nearly 60,000 bombers of all sizes. Allied industry and research also led to new types of bombs, including, ultimately, the atomic bombs that killed 140,000 people at Hiroshima and 80,000 at Nagasaki, most of them civilian.

Of course, civilians had suffered terribly in wars of previous eras, but they had never been targets for extermination on the levels of the victims of Nazi Germany and Imperial Japan. Furthermore, the increased speed, scale, and scope of the war put civilians in the middle of (or below) the new weapons of war much more often than ever before. The end result, both intended and accidental, was a tremendous increase in civilian casualties. One study of orphans estimated that 13,000,000 children had *both* parents killed during the war.[1]

The other important change involved the dramatically increased role of women (so much so that we must change the sub-heading above). Of course, the intentional targeting of civilians mentioned above included women (and for that matter, children as well). But more fundamentally, women took on military roles and responsibilities as never before. In World War I, women had worked in military-related industries and served in nursing and ambulance corps. But in World War II they did so in numbers so unprecedented that many domestic conservatives worried that the fabric of their societies was coming undone. Between 1939 and 1943 the British workforce added 2,160,000 female workers and nearly 1,000,000 more women joined the armed services or civil defense. About the same number of women served in the Soviet armed forces, while at the same time Soviet women came, by 1943, to make up fifty-seven per cent of the civilian industrial workforce and seventy-three per cent of the agricultural workforce.

Most military women served in "auxiliaries" designed to concentrate women into traditionally female occupations like clerking and secretarial jobs. The names of some like the United States Navy's WAVES (Women Accepted for Volunteer Emergency Service) reveal the temporary and subordinate nature that most planners envisioned for them. Some, like the British Navy's WRNS (Women's Royal Navy Service, pronounced "wrens"), and United States' WASP (Women's Airforce Service Pilots) fought for years to attain official military status. Still, they increasingly performed "male" jobs including non-combat piloting and anti-aircraft duties.

Soviet women entered combat services in the largest concentrations, albeit only as a temporary expedient. They became snipers, tank drivers, and combat pilots. The Germans dubbed one group of particularly effective female bomber pilots the "Night Witches." British and American women, while rarely in direct combat, performed the dangerous job of ferrying new (and often unreliable) planes from their factories to bases. Even the Germans, always reluctant to put women in "male" military jobs, nevertheless had a female test pilot who flew the V-1 before it was converted into an unmanned weapon. Women also played critical roles in partisan warfare and resistance groups in France, Italy, Yugoslavia, and elsewhere. The Germans deported 10,000 French women to concentration camps for resistance activities; only 500 survived.

The majority of the men who served entered their nation's military via conscription. The totality of World War II, combined with the lower percentage of the great powers' population who were needed to grow food, meant that armies became vastly larger than they had ever been before. Conscription was the only way to rationally access men without severely disrupting domestic economies. Whereas in 1939 the United States, Britain, the Soviet Union, Germany, and Japan had a combined 5,600,000 men under arms, by 1944 they had 45,400,000. The United States alone had nearly 15,000,000. Training these men and women required an unprecedented array of schools and development centers. The complex technology and logistics required to move men and material around the world inspired a vast array of non-combat specializations. The ratio of men and women who fought to men and women who supported them (the so-called "tooth-to-tail" ratio) tipped in favor of the latter for the first time in history.

Military leadership also changed its focus. The revolution in communications technology, especially the wireless radio and effective field telephones, allowed ground commanders to lead from the front. Many of the war's most famous generals, like the American George Patton, the British Bernard Montgomery, and the German Erwin Rommel eschewed the "château generalship" of World War I and led from, or quite near, the front lines. They became heroes both for their leadership and for personalizing a war that engulfed the lives of millions of men, women, and children around the world.

The machines

Many of the machines of World War II were based on technologies and ideas developed in World War I, but few of them would have been recognizable to the men of 1918. The American Liberty aircraft engine was a great feat of engineering for World War I, but its 400 horsepower was absolutely dwarfed by the 1,700 horsepower of the North American P-51D fighter introduced in 1944. To cite another example, the fearsome German Gotha bomber of World War I had a maximum speed of eighty-eight miles per hour, a range of 522 miles, and carried 1,100 pounds of bombs. The American B-29A of World War II, by contrast, flew 342 miles per hour, had an amazing range of 4,100 miles and carried a maximum bomb load of 20,000 pounds. World War II also saw the introduction of entirely new weapons systems including jet aircraft, rockets, and, most radically, atomic weapons. Both in terms of the tremendous evolution of existing weapons systems and the revolution in others, World War II represents a true watershed in military technology.

This level of technological change represents the confluence of three important world history themes: the industrial revolution; the growth of state power; and the emergence of the United States as a global power. The first two themes date to the eighteenth century, but reached their apex during World War II. The national crises occasioned by the war resulted in the conversion of consumer industries, like automobiles and electronics, to military production. This concentration of economic resources into military hardware meant that weapons, transportation systems, and other necessities could be produced in quantities that would have been unthinkable just a few years earlier.

Similarly, state power and the ability to manage economic resources also increased. Fascism and Soviet-style communism both operated (at least theoretically) under the philosophy of centralized control of economics. The Soviet system especially operated under the centralized command system. Even the western democracies increased their levels of control over industrial production, though the Americans used a capitalist profit model (called the "cost-plus" system, designed to guarantee profits to civilian manufacturers) to encourage production.

The results were astounding. Despite the disruptions caused by air attacks and occupations, the five major powers (Britain, the United States, Germany, the Soviet Union, and Japan) increased aircraft production from 36,940 planes in 1939 to 231,066 in 1944, major naval vessel production from ninety-three in 1939 to 3,093 in 1944, and tank production from 5,210 in 1939 to 74,029 in 1944. These astonishing levels of industrial production provided the tools for a war of unimagined cruelty.

The United States had several important advantages in the field of industrial production. Alone among the great powers, the United States suffered from neither enemy occupation nor from strategic bombing. The United States also had access to abundant raw materials at home and favorable trade terms with Latin America with which to acquire more. The United States Army also made a controversial decision to limit itself to ninety divisions (of approximately 15,000 men each); this "ninety division gamble" freed a greater percentage of men for industry than was the case for the other major combatants. American women joined the work force by the hundreds of thousands as did many African-Americans who moved into northern and western cities in large numbers to take factory jobs.

The United States' role as "the Arsenal of Democracy" (to use President Franklin Roosevelt's famous phrase) was critical to Allied victory. Indeed, the United States was so productive that it was able to equip itself and still provide vast quantities of critical goods to its allies. Through a series of agreements collectively known as the Lend-Lease program, the United States distributed close to $50,000,000,000 worth of aid to thirty-eight countries. Great Britain (which received almost half of the total aid) and the Soviet Union were the primary recipients, but China and Australia also benefited tremendously. To take just one case (and not even the largest), the United States provided the USSR with 34,000,000 sets of uniforms; 15,000,000 pairs of boots; 350,000 tons of explosives; 3,000,000 tons of gasoline; untold millions of tons of food; 12,000 railroad cars; 375,000 trucks; and 50,000 jeeps. Lend-Lease also helped nations like Brazil (which received $366,000,000 in aid) and Mexico (which received $39,000,000) escape the Great Depression and become important regional economic nexuses.

The United States was also the production center for many of the war's most effective weapons systems. The aircraft carrier gave navies long-distance striking power. American faith in the carriers was born partly out of necessity; by a stroke of incredible good fortune the only three Pacific Fleet carriers were at sea when the Japanese struck Pearl Harbor and sank or severely damaged all eight of the Pacific Fleet battleships. In 1942, the United States introduced the *Essex* class carrier. It eventually built twenty-four of them; no other nation ever built more than seven ships of similar size in the same class. Each *Essex* carrier could carry ninety-one airplanes. Carriers radically changed the nature of naval warfare. In 1942, for the first time in history, two fleets (the American and Japanese at the Battle of Coral Sea) fought one another without the ships ever seeing one another. Carrier-based aviation fought the entire action.

Non-weapons technologies also played critical roles. After the fall of Poland in 1939, British researchers acquired an Enigma machine, used by the Germans to write a code that they thought was too complex to be broken. But the British, using a top-secret sta 10,000, did break it. The intelligence they received, codenamed ULTRA, proved absolutely vital to the British in several theaters of the war and played a key role in Britain's ability to defeat repeated air attacks by the German Ai   during the Battle of Britain in 1940 and 1941.

The United States also benefited from intelligence, codenamed MAGIC, deciphered from the Japanese. MAGIC allowed the Americans to make a reliable educated guess that the Japanese were planning to attack Midway Island in summer, 1942. The Americans knew that the Japanese were planning to attack a target they had codenamed AI. An American officer, acting on a hunch that AI was Midway Island, sent a message that he knew the Japanese could intercept. The message stated that Midway's fresh water system was not functioning properly. Shortly thereafter, MAGIC deciphered a Japanese message saying that AI was out of fresh water. By the time of the Japanese attack, American cryptographers had decoded the entire Japanese plan. Armed with that information, the United States Navy was able to win the battle, despite having inferior numbers, by concentrating its forces around Midway rather than dispersing them to cover the entire theater. Code breaking and ciphering machines provided an invaluable advantage to the Allies. Neither the Japanese nor the Germans enjoyed anywhere near the same level of success in this arena.

All of the major powers had access to Radar (Radio Detection and Ranging) technology during the war, but Great Britain excelled. Its 1940 discovery of the cavity magnetron led to the 1943 Anglo-American introduction of highly effective centimetric radar systems. British superiority in radar technology allowed the Royal Air Force to track incoming German planes and send interceptors. It also allowed for more efficient navigation systems for British bombers attacking German industrial centers. Japan was especially hamstrung by the lack of effective radar, all the more so because of the inability of the Japanese army and navy to agree on a system for combining their two networks.

World War II also saw the introduction (and the only two war time uses) of the atomic bomb, a weapon that, as we will see, radically altered concepts of military strategy and operations. The flights of German-Jewish scientist Albert Einstein and Italian scientist Enrico Fermi (whose wife was Jewish) from Europe in 1938 marked the start of Allied research. Einstein warned the British and American governments that German scientists had split the atom, a critical prerequisite for building an atomic weapon. In 1942, after American entry into the war, Britain, the United States, and Canada created the highly-secret Manhattan Project to coordinate all research and activity on nuclear energy. The project eventually cost $2,000,000,000, most of it American, and required tremendous coordination and research. The construction of one research complex (at Hanford, Washington) was at the time the largest construction project in American history. Another (at Oak Ridge, Tennessee) was then the largest building in the country.

In the end, the Allies had a superweapon that made an invasion of the Japanese home islands unnecessary. While the motivations behind the use of the bomb (especially the second bomb, dropped on Nagasaki) remain subjects of historical debate, few on the Allied side in 1945 felt anything but joy and relief that the war was over. Unbeknownst to the Americans and British, however, Soviet spies had acquired vital intelligence about the atomic bomb. In 1949, well ahead of American estimates, the Soviets exploded their own atomic bomb, adding radioactive fuel to the expanding Cold War.

The battles

Unlike the stalemate of trench warfare that characterized World War I, the technologies of World War II led to battles that covered miles of ground and/or water and moved quickly. Many of the new technologies and doctrines allowed for battles to occur with lightning speed. Indeed, Germany's war doctrine of 1939 and 1940, Blitzkrieg (lightning war), aptly described the speed and pace of much of the war. Germany, like the other great powers, had been traumatized by the senseless waste of the trenches in World War I. Blitzkrieg was Germany's answer for eliminating the trenches. They designed Blitzkrieg around rapid movement by mechanized infantry (although in fact most men continued to march), airplanes, and tanks, all connected by radio. This system worked well against smaller nations close to Germany's border such as Poland, Holland, and Norway.

The French, whose mentality was much more defensive, were at an important disadvantage against this new type of warfare. France had responded to the horrors of the trenches by building a formidable line of defenses named for Minister of War André Maginot, a veteran of Verdun in 1916. But France left their border with Belgium unguarded, leaving an important opening for the German Blitzkrieg. This German system, so effective against neighbors, proved ill-suited to enemies protected by water, like Britain, or those far away, like the Soviet Union.

Water, thousands of square miles of it, was Japan's most serious problem. To solve it, they turned to modern technology, selectively adapted from the west. The Imperial Japanese Navy had carefully studied a dramatic 1940 British carrier attack on the Italian naval base at Taranto in the Italian "heel." In one surprise stroke the British changed the naval balance of power in the Mediterranean as the Japanese were hoping to do in the Pacific. Aircraft carriers allowed the Japanese navy to get close enough to Pearl Harbor to launch 350 planes without the Americans being able to respond effectively. The result was a punishing blow to the battleships of the American Pacific Fleet. Three days later, Japanese carrier-based planes sank two of Britain's prized surface ships, the *Prince of Wales* and the *Repulse*, leaving the South China Sea wide open for Japanese expansion. Surface ships thereafter acted without air cover at their own risk.

Paratroopers, initially devised by the Russians in the 1920s, added another new dimension to warfare. First used in combat by the Germans in Norway and Holland in 1940, paratroopers could add speed and shock by landing on or behind enemy lines. Because they have to jump into battle with all of the supplies they will need, they are normally "light" infantry, meaning that they need to be relieved or resupplied quickly. It also means that they are vulnerable to "heavier" units. In an airborne attack over the island of Crete in 1941, German paratroopers landed too close to British Commonwealth positions, causing such high casualties that the German high command suspended their use of paratroops.

Ironically, the Allies learned from the German disaster and developed a doctrine of landing airborne troops away from enemy formations, then reforming the units to act as regular infantry behind enemy lines. This approach proved to be critically important to the success of the D-Day operation of June, 1944 (see the introduction). Of course, airborne operations were quite risky. Later in 1944 many of the same men who had parachuted over Normandy dropped over Holland as part of a bold British plan code-named MARKET GARDEN. This time, the men unintentionally dropped directly on top of two elite German SS Panzer (tank) units. Half of the British 1st

Airborne Division became prisoners of war. The American 82nd and 101st Airborne Divisions lost 3,500 men.

In the Pacific Theater, neither the Americans nor the Japanese were fully prepared for the challenges of war in the inhospitable islands of the tropics. Despite the pre-war rushes of the European powers to colonize, many of the islands that would become hotly contested were little-known to outsiders. Neither side had accurate maps nor did they understand the cultures of the people living there. Japanese torture and terror proved less effective than American goods and money in winning the loyalty of locals in these islands. Native "coast watchers" and porters provided vital intelligence, scouting, and labor to the Americans. Both sides suffered terribly from disease and experienced significant supply problems as a result of the tremendous distances involved (Pearl Harbor is more than 5,000 miles from Manila).

A clash of cultures, races, and battlefield doctrines turned the Pacific War into one of terrifying brutality. Since Japan's "opening" to the west in 1853 it had modernized its military to the point that in many ways it closely resembled its American, British, and Australian foes. Still, the proximity that jungle fighting required and the near-fanatical resistance to surrender (and, as a result, their lack of respect for prisoners of war) on the part of the Japanese turned the "island hopping" campaigns of the war into what one historian called a "war without mercy." One survey found that forty-eight per cent of United States Army troops agreed with the statement "I would really like to kill a Japanese" whereas only nine per cent felt the same way about killing a German soldier.[2]

The Japanese and Germans found it impossible to keep up with Allied production capacity and the operational flexibility that such production provided. Over the course of the war, the United States and Britain built more than 46,000 landing craft along with a vast array of support ships to protect and supply them. Although these craft had to be divided among several theaters, they gave the Allies the flexibility to land men behind enemy lines. This ability allowed the Allies to constantly keep the Japanese army and navy off balance in the Pacific as well as conduct major amphibious operations in North Africa in 1942, Italy in January, 1944 (where the small town of Anzio temporarily became the world's fourth largest port), northern France (D-Day) in June, then southern France in August. The United States Marine Corps had been intensively studying the problems of amphibious warfare, including the failed British landing at Galipolli in 1915, since 1933. Their training, plus the landing and support ships of the United States Navy, played a key role in the defeat of Japan.

All of these technologies and doctrines came together by 1944. In Normandy, France on 6 June, 1944 23,400 paratroopers landed before dawn to cut German supply lines while 7,000 ships (supported by massive air assaults) bombarded German positions and landed 75,000 men. Within one month, the Allies had placed an incredible 850,000 men, 148,000 vehicles, and 570,000 tons of supplies in France. Less than a year later the Allies repeated the feat with different forces halfway around the world at Okinawa.

World War II saw warfare being fought by all classes of weapons in all kinds of terrains. Soldiers endured jungle warfare in places like Burma and the islands of the south Pacific; desert warfare in North Africa; urban warfare from Berlin to Manila; arctic warfare in Finland and mountain warfare in Norway and the Caucasus. Submarines patrolled the waters of all of the world's oceans and airplanes made global reach a possibility. After 1945 no place on the globe was immune to the worldwide nature of military operations.

Legacies

In large measure, the world wars were merely a military manifestation of the increasing globalism that had been characterizing world history for more than a century. The same technologies that facilitated global trade and imperialism made war on a global scale possible. But the revolutionary changes in speed and scope made these interactions an entirely new phenomenon. This era of "military globalism" continued into the post-war period. Military operations and alliances were now cross-continental and truly global.

A second important legacy involves the clear and notable decline of western Europe as a center of world power. The two world wars sapped much of those nations' military and financial energies. By the middle of the war, the British had been forced to recognize that they were junior partners in their alliance with the United States. France was militarily, politically, and psychologically shaken by the four-year German occupation, Italy was in tatters, Germany was divided and occupied by the victorious allies. All faced staggering financial problems, severely damaged industrial infrastructures, and exhausted populations.

One clear consequence of the "decline of the west" was the weakening of Europe's grip on their colonial empires. Even before the war's conclusion, nationalist groups began efforts to use the war to achieve their own independence. In India in 1942, the Indian National Congress adopted a "Quit India Resolution," that called on the British to leave. Ho Chi Minh had similar plans to use the chaos of the war to achieve independence for Vietnam. He proclaimed the Democratic Republic of Vietnam in Hanoi just two weeks after the Japanese surrender, directly challenging French desires to reoccupy Indochina after the war.

Another clear consequence of the decline of western Europe was the emergence of the two "superpowers," the United States and the Soviet Union. The alliance between the two nations during the war had always been a marriage of convenience, fueled by a common need to defeat Germany. Even before the end of the war, however, mutual suspicions and long-standing conflicts between the two had soured relations. Some historians have argued that the United States used the atomic bombs against Japan in part to warn Russia that the United States possessed such weapons.

The atomic bomb remains the war's most terrifying legacy. Research on the bombs during the war had been so secret that American Vice-President Harry Truman had to be told about their existence upon his accession to the presidency in April, 1945. Even most of the scientists, confined to working on small pieces of the project, had little understanding of the larger picture. No one knew exactly what effect the new weapons would have on the future of warfare, but it was soon obvious that mankind possessed a weapon many thousands of times greater than any that had previously existed. It was equally obvious that research on such weapons would continue, both in the United States and inside the laboratories of the Soviet Union as well.

Notes

1 See Williamson Murray and Allan Millett, *A War to be Won: Fighting the Second World War* (Cambridge: Harvard University Press, 2000), p. 553.
2 Ronald Spector, *Eagle Against the Sun* (New York: Vintage Press), Chapter 18.

Further reading

World War II has generated a terrific and broad-based literature. Take this list as a general starting point. Good surveys include John Keegan, *The Second World War* (New York, Penguin, 1989); Martin Gilbert, *The Second World War* (New York: Henry Holt, 1989); and Williamson Murray and Allan Millett, *A War to be Won: Fighting the Second World War* (Cambridge: Harvard University Press, 2000). Among the best analytic studies are: Richard Overy, *Why the Allies Won* (New York: Norton, 1995); Omer Bartov, *Hitler's Army: Soldiers, Nazis, and War in the Third Reich* (New York: Oxford University Press, 1991); Michael Doubler, *Closing with the Enemy: How GIs Fought the War in Europe* (Lawrence: University Press of Kansas, 1994); and John Dower, *War Without Mercy: Race and Power in the Pacific War* (New York: Pantheon Books, 1986). Excellent readable accounts of individual campaigns include Cornelius Ryan's *The Longest Day* (New York: Touchstone, 1959) on D-Day and Antony Beevor's *Stalingrad: The Fateful Siege, 1942–1943* (New York: Penguin, 1998).

Chapter 7

The Cold War and beyond

Dien Bien Phu, 1953–1954

In a remote corner of northwestern Vietnam, near the Chinese and Laotian borders, the French had staked their hopes on retaining their colonial possessions in Southeast Asia. Beginning in November, 1953 the French had converted the valley known as Dien Bien Phu into a fortified position into which they hoped to draw Viet Minh guerrilla forces and destroy them. Fifteen thousand French and French Foreign Legion troops built nine fortified strong points and two airstrips. Since 1947, the French presence in Vietnam had been steadily weakened in the face of anti-imperial forces, most notably the Viet Minh. The French believed that their position at Dien Bien Phu was too strong for the Vietnamese to take and would be an important base for cutting off supply routes and returning French hegemony to the area.

The French badly misjudged the resolve of the Viet Minh and their military leader, Vo Nguyen Giap. His men dragged 200 artillery pieces, including Chinese-made anti-aircraft artillery, through the jungle and into high-ground positions above the valley around the northeastern-most fortification, named Béatrice. Giap attacked on 14 March 1954 and seized Béatrice in a matter of hours. Two other strong points guarding the northern airstrip fell within seventy-two hours. Viet Minh guns could then be put in position to attack French aircraft attempting to land at the airstrips or trying to airdrop supplies. The Viet Minh destroyed or damaged 169 of the 420 French airplanes available to support Dien Bien Phu. Without air support, the French garrison was cut off from resupply. Giap also directed attacks at French positions across Vietnam to prevent French reinforcements from reaching the garrison by land. The Viet Minh, on the other hand, operating in an area friendly to them, could call on the civilian population for food and be assured that their own lines of communication were relatively safe.

One by one, the Viet Minh attacked the French strong points using human wave tactics that were extremely costly, but wore down the French defenders and their remaining supplies. The opening of an international conference in Geneva, Switzerland in April to determine the future of Vietnam raised the stakes for both sides. France's most powerful ally, the United States, ruled out air strikes to relieve the garrison, though the possibility that the Americans might intervene further heightened the anxiety around Dien Bien Phu. The Viet Minh changed tactics to a combination of frontal attacks, artillery, and mines. In May, the Viet Minh launched a final assault on the tenacious French garrison. Out of ammunition and out of food, the French surrendered on 7 May. Virtually the entire 15,000 man French garrison was dead, wounded, or captured. The Viet Minh had lost 25,000 men and women, but the fall of Dien Bien Phu led the French to sign the Geneva Accords in July and end their colonial presence in Southeast Asia.

The French tried desperately to combat Viet Minh guerrillas with conventional military forces. They were stunned by the ability of such guerrillas to neutralize or counter virtually all of their technological advantages. As the Americans would later do in the same part of the world, the French vastly underestimated the morale and capability of their guerrilla foes and greatly overestimated their own military ability and national will to fight such a force. Dien Bien Phu ranks as one of the greatest victories for a guerrilla force over a conventional one. It virtually ended one Vietnam war and set the stage for a second.

It is useful to think in terms of two types of warfare in this period: symmetrical and asymmetrical. In symmetrical wars, the opposing sides have militaries that share a basic organizational structure, have a reasonably equivalent level of technology, and use similar doctrines. In asymmetrical wars, one side possesses seemingly overwhelming advantages in these areas. Because of the dynamism of guerrillas in the twentieth century, the supposed advantages of wealthier powers in asymmetrical wars have not always produced victory. As the Viet Minh at Dien Bien Phu demonstrated, guerrilla forces found ways to compensate for the apparent disadvantages they held against their wealthier, and seemingly stronger, foes.

The men and women

As the Dien Bien Phu example demonstrates, the post-World War II period is in many respects the age of the guerrilla. Guerrillas took on many forms in this period, but they shared three traits: the need to fight with limited resources, normally against a force armed with modern weapons; a nationalist or ideological commitment to fighting that normally exceeded the level of commitment of their enemies; and significant levels of support from local communities. This connection to local communities provided food, intelligence, and other forms of support (sometimes coerced) that were critical in counterbalancing the money and supplies of larger powers.

Guerrillas were not new to warfare. Julius Caesar complained of the difficulty of subduing guerrillas in Britain. Spanish guerrillas dogged Napoleon. Boer guerrillas harassed the British in the Boer Wars. T. E. Lawrence used guerrilla tactics to great effect in the Middle East during World War I. Before the 1950s, however, guerrilla success was the exception rather than the rule. More often than not, guerrillas only won when they acted as support units to allied conventional units (as in the Spanish case) or as distractions to the enemy's other efforts (as in T. E. Lawrence's case). But in the Cold War period guerrillas experienced unprecedented levels of success.

The rise of the guerrilla is consistent with a key theme of the post-World War II period: the decline of imperialism. The world wars left the European colonizing powers militarily and financially weaker, especially in relation to the United States and the Soviet Union. Neither of the new "superpowers" was interested in sustaining imperialism, at least not on the British or French model. In some cases, notably in India, the European power, in this case Great Britain, decided not to fight to reassert colonial power. In others, notably Indochina, Algeria, and Malaysia, France and Britain attempted to reestablish their old colonial hegemony. Although the world wars had left Europe weaker, France and Britain still held out the potential to bring enormous resources to bear, especially after the Marshall Plan and other economic recovery efforts began to bear fruit. Those people wishing to resist recolonization therefore had to search for military means that were relatively less demanding of resources.

In part, the success of guerrilla forces was a function of the anti-imperial energies created by decolonization. The most famous examples are the Vietnamese forces that resisted Japanese imperialism during World War II, overthrew a French attempt to recolonize Indochina from 1947 to 1954, defeated the Americans from 1965 to 1973, then fought off a Chinese invasion in 1979. In all four cases, they faced armies with much more highly sophisticated military technology. They won in large part because they held fiercely to ideals of independence and were willing to fight for them longer than any of their foes were willing to oppose them.

Guerrilla success was also a function of the superpowers' obsession with each other. The United States and the Soviet Union amassed large nuclear and conventional forces, developed sophisticated doctrines, and formed global alliances with the intention of deterring or fighting one another. To their surprise and dismay, they discovered that such forces and alliances were ill-designed to fight smaller, less technologically sophisticated groups in asymmetrical wars. The United States' nuclear arsenal, its fleet of attack submarines, and its armored forces were of little use in the jungles of Vietnam. The Soviet Union discovered the same problem in the deserts of Afghanistan soon afterward. On a smaller scale, the pattern also held in the Middle East. Israel's sophisticated and highly modern military defeated much larger Arab conventional forces in 1956, 1967, and 1973. When the same force tried to fight the Palestinian *Intifada*, a popular uprising, Israel found that it could not easily bring its military advantages to bear. The British have experienced similar problems in using their regular forces to defeat the Irish Republican Army.

Guerrillas forced more technologically sophisticated opponents into low-intensity situations where military technology could not be used with its full impact. They rarely opened themselves up to the kinds of large-scale battles that their opponents were accustomed to fighting. When they did, as in the Vietnamese Tet Offensive of 1968, the results were often disastrous. After three years of guerrilla war against the Americans, the Vietnamese gambled on a full offensive during the Vietnamese New Year, known as Tet. In effect, by exposing their units in conventional battle, the Vietnamese turned an asymmetrical war into a symmetrical one. Initially, the Vietnamese surprised the Americans and scored dramatic successes, but once the Americans recovered, they were able to use the full power of their weapons systems on the exposed (and now symmetrical) Vietnamese. Vietnamese guerrilla and regular forces suffered terrible casualties, but Tet made Americans question the value of the war, and is normally considered the most important turning point of the war.

Guerrillas normally preferred to fight when enemy advantages could be reduced or neutralized. Chinese leader Mao Tse-Tung's ideas on guerrilla strategy, influenced by the ancient Chinese thinker Sun Tzu, were widely read, modified, and implemented throughout the world. His principles involved luring the enemy deep into one's own territory to stress his logistical system as much as possible and to put him in unfamiliar terrain. Guerrillas could then attack quickly, inflict damage, and fade into the countryside. Attacking at close range could also help to negate the enemy's superiority of firepower. Only when the enemy had thus been reduced in strength did Mao advocate engaging in conventional warfare.

Guerrillas therefore fought a low-intensity, but total, form of warfare. When successful, this form of warfare proved to be remarkably resilient, with guerrillas often willing to fight for years or decades if necessary. This commitment stretched the popular and military will of larger powers, for whom wars against guerrillas were normally a side show. To the United States and the Soviet Union, in Vietnam and Afghanistan respectively, the wars were limited. To the Vietnamese and the Afghanis, of course, they were total. In Kenya, by contrast, the British were willing to commit enough resources to outwait the insurgents and win the war.

In Africa, guerrillas won bloody victories in Eritrea, Ethiopia, Uganda, Rwanda, the Congo, and elsewhere. Some scholars contend that African guerrillas are normally more susceptible to tribalism and warlordism than are guerrillas in Asia and Latin America. These same scholars also argue that African guerrillas are less disciplined, less formally organized, and have more often resorted to terror than their counterparts elsewhere. Therefore, guerrilla warfare in Africa has produced much higher death totals than might be expected given the combatants' relatively primitive weapons. Conventional armies, like Portugal's in Angola and the United States' in Mogadishu, were frustrated by their inability to enforce their will on such groups despite tremendous advantages in discipline and technology.

Of course, not all warriors were guerrillas. Many nations continued the traditional pattern of large forces-in-being. These forces were arranged within several competing alliance systems, the most important being the North Atlantic Treaty Organization (NATO, formed in 1949) dominated by the United States, and the Warsaw Pact (formed in 1955), dominated by the Soviet Union. As a result, the military forces of the alliances were designed to deter and fight each other. This mission required large armies and, in most cases, conscription. The draft became unpopular in the United States in the late 1960s as a result of its connection to the Vietnam War. Critics alleged that class and race inequities forced a disproportionate share of the nation's military burden onto the poor and members of minority groups. The United States abandoned conscription in the early 1970s. In Europe, the apparent end of the Cold War in 1989 led to increasing pressures to abandon conscription. It has been phased out in most European nations since.

The post-World War II period has also marked the rising participation of women in military affairs, in both guerrilla armies and conventional ones. In part this change has been a reflection of women's widening opportunities in civilian society, especially in the west. By the end of the twentieth century, women had taken on important roles in all of the western militaries. They are now admitted to all western military academies, can become fighter pilots in all western air forces, and have achieved senior rank. Women are now a part of the once ultra-macho French Foreign Legion as well. The only military jobs normally closed to them are submarine service, ground combat, and special operations, though even there challenges have tried to push the limits.

Israel is perhaps the most famous example. Both a westernized society with opportunities for women in civilian life and a society with compelling defense needs, Israel subjects both men and women to military conscription. The tradition of female participation in Israeli defense dates back to the formation of the state. In 1949, five women commanded combat units. This tradition notwithstanding, gender segregation continues. Women are separated into an organization whose acronym is Chen (Chail Nashim or women's corps), which also translates as "charm." Women can also obtain exemptions from military service much more easily than men can. Still, the Israeli Defense Forces include women in several important positions and in all Israeli wars, women have served in front-line combat units.

Women's roles in guerrilla and non-western armies have expanded as well. The *Sendero Luminoso* or "Shining Path" rebels of Peru have almost always had a female second-in-command. In 1992, forty per cent of its members were women. By one estimate, anywhere from thirty-three per cent to fifty per cent of Viet Cong (the name that the Viet Minh took on in the 1960s) members during the Vietnam War were female. At one point, forty per cent of Viet Cong regimental commanders were women. In Africa, women have also played critical roles; in one famous example, a Zimbabwean commander led troops that fought off a Rhodesian attack just two days after giving birth. In most of the developing world, women's military roles are less a reflection of desires for social and political equity (as is often the case in the west), and more a function of what historian Linda Grant De Pauw calls "grim necessity."[1]

The machines

The most powerful weapons of this period were, fortunately, never used. America's nuclear monopoly after World War II lasted just four years. In 1949, the Soviet Union exploded its first atomic bomb, prompting the Americans to begin research into much deadlier hydrogen bombs. The United States completed its hydrogen bomb program with a successful detonation in 1952. The Soviets kept pace, detonating their own hydrogen device just a year later. Nuclear proliferation spread to other great powers, with Great Britain exploding its first nuclear device in 1952 (followed by the explosion of its first hydrogen bomb in 1957). The British program was closely tied to that of the United States. France's was not. The French, looking for a military deterrent independent of the United States and NATO became the world's fourth nuclear power in 1960. China's first atomic bomb was exploded in 1964, its first hydrogen bomb three years later. Today, it is widely accepted that at the very least, South Africa, Israel, Pakistan, and India either have nuclear weapons or possess the potential to build them quickly.

The means for delivering a nuclear device also developed widely. Larger and more powerful jet bombers, like the massive American B-52, provided the ability to disperse the delivery capability. So, too, did modern submarines, whose nuclear power plants provided nearly unlimited range. Such submarines are capable of launching nuclear missiles from a spot just off the coast of an enemy power. Intercontinental Ballistic Missiles provided another option. Eventually, nuclear missiles became capable of carrying multiple warheads. In their race to keep pace with each other and their search for the upper hand, the superpowers developed the ability to destroy the planet several times over, defeating the point of traditional military strategy. A military force that destroyed the world could not, obviously, help the state pursue political and economic goals.

The evident horrors of nuclear warfare thus led to an emphasis on deterrence rather than warfare at the nuclear level. In essence, the goal of the nuclear powers was to possess enough power to deter an enemy from launching a nuclear attack. The Americans and Soviets developed forces that they believed were sufficient to survive an enemy first strike and still retain enough power to annihilate the other side. Such strategic thinking led to the most appropriate acronym in military history, MAD or Mutually Assured Destruction. If each side possessed the power to survive an attack and still destroy the other side, the thinking went, no one would start a war.

Such thinking was safe in the theoretical world, but the sheer power of the world's nuclear arms meant that a single decision, or even an accident, could lead to a war capable of destroying all life. The margin of error in these cases was extremely small. In a few instances, most notably during the Cuban Missile Crisis of 1962, deterrence seemed quite shaky indeed. The United States met Soviet attempts to deploy missiles in Cuba with a naval and air blockade of the island. Both the American and Soviet militaries went on full alert. Eventually the two sides negotiated an end to the crisis (the Soviets agreed not to deploy missiles in Cuba and the United States removed its missiles from Turkey), but it demonstrated how precarious deterrence could be. In 1963, the two superpowers established a direct "hot line" between the White House and the Kremlin in hopes of avoiding future crises, though both militaries went on full alert again during the Arab-Israeli War of 1973.

On the conventional level, advancements in computer technology and satellites provided the ability to produce a new generation of weapons. Precision Guided Munitions (PGMs) or so-called "smart" weapons can be delivered with little or no risk to human operators. PGMs can take the form of laser guided bombs dropped from an airplane or cruise missiles launched from hundreds of miles away and capable of flying underneath radar systems. Cruise missiles have on-board radar systems that are linked to satellite navigation systems to direct them onto a specific target. Advocates of such weapons praise the ability of PGMs to reduce civilian casualties (called "collateral damage") by more precisely striking specified targets. A video image of an American bomb falling down an Iraqi air shaft received much television time during the Persian Gulf War. Critics allege that such weapons remove the individual from warfare, making war take on the air of a sanitary video game.

The vast array of sophisticated military weaponry developed by wealthy nations rarely proved to be applicable to low-intensity guerrilla warfare. As one American observer noted of the Vietnam War, the United States seemed to be trying to kill a fly with a sledgehammer. The weapons of guerrillas tended to be similar to those of warriors from earlier ages, most commonly rifles, primitive explosives, or even machetes. The guerrilla's lack of advanced systems removed the need for complex logistical and support systems. The relative simplicity of the guerrilla system also made it easier for peasants and other people untrained in modern military organization to participate in warfare.

Advancements in computer technology also revolutionized military organization and communications. Computers and sophisticated data management techniques allowed for greater control over ever larger forces. Not all of the consequences of computerization were expected or beneficial. Computers had the unexpected outcome of emphasizing information that could be quantified at the expense of those factors, like morale, that could not. The Americans therefore judged their success in Vietnam on "body counts" and the quest for a "crossover point" at which Americans were supposedly killing Vietnamese guerrillas faster than they could be replaced. Such a system rewarded units that killed the enemy, leading many officers to exaggerate or fabricate body counts.

American units often reported all dead Vietnamese as enemy soldiers, further distorting the statistics upon which American decision makers relied.

Although it is now largely a civilian resource, the internet was initially designed as a military communications device. Decentralized as it is, the internet would theoretically allow military computer networks to remain connected together even in the event that an enemy strike disabled several points along the network. Without its computer networks, a modern military system effectively has to operate without its ears and eyes. As such, communications centers have become important targets to military planners (guerrilla forces normally lack such centers, further frustrating those who fight them). Technicians have become as important to military operations as soldiers. Indeed, the two roles have in many cases become synonymous.

Computers also mean that warfare can now be conducted from a much greater distance. Missile operators can reach almost any target in the world with the turn of a key or the push of a button. Midair refueling technology has allowed combat aircraft to have a nearly unlimited range. American pilots can now take off from bases in the middle of the United States, strike a target in Serbia with PGMs, and return home without ever having landed or achieved visual contact with the target.

Advances in military medicine have greatly improved the ability of modern militaries to care for their wounded. Sophisticated militaries can quite literally bring an entire hospital into a theater of war if necessary. Helicopters allow militaries to evacuate wounded directly off a battlefield to a fabricated hospital or a fully provisioned hospital ship nearby. As a result, thousands of soldiers now survive wounds that in earlier periods would have killed them. In Korea and Vietnam the American died-of-wounds rate dropped to as low as three per cent. Disease rates have also dropped as field sanitation has improved, new medicines have been introduced, and commanders learned to take preventive medicine more seriously. These improvements do not mean, of course, that combat has become any less dangerous, just that military medicine has dramatically improved.

The development of weapons in the post-World War II period reinforces two important themes. First, during the Cold War, the two superpowers produced weapons systems capable of inflicting unprecedented damage. By the 1980s each side had developed a triad of delivery systems (airplanes, submarines, and missiles) capable of striking any target in the world with a nuclear weapon within thirty minutes. After the collapse of the Soviet Union, the United States assumed the mantle of the world's lone superpower. The Soviet nuclear program decentralized among its constituent republics, making new nations like Ukraine, Belarus, and Kazakhstan important nuclear powers in their own right until arrangements could be made to decommission or "deproliferate" their stockpiles.

Second, despite the enormous complexity in weapons systems in the developed world, the developing world remained militarily dynamic.

Guerrillas frequently fought long and hard enough to force more powerful foes to stop fighting. The military advantages of the United States, Russia, and western Europe should not be read as evidence of their ability to enforce policy at will. Moreover, regional powers like India, Egypt, South Africa, and Brazil were still able to carve out important regional hegemony. More recently, concerns over the proliferation of so-called "weapons of mass destruction" have led advanced nations to fear the spread of nuclear, biological, and chemical capability to states like Iraq, North Korea, and others. The world remains a dangerous place.

The battles

The great battle that NATO and the Warsaw Pact planned for and feared, a major clash in central or western Europe, never occurred. The awesome nuclear power that the two sides amassed deterred a conventional war for fear of the consequence of escalation. Nevertheless, the Cold War played an important military role across the globe as the United States and the Soviet Union fought one another through client states. Each side armed governments friendly to itself and funded guerrilla opponents of unfriendly governments. As a result, armies in the Middle East, Asia, Africa, and Central America obtained the money and resources both to start wars and to sustain them. Although they were not decisive, Soviet supplies of surface-to-air missile batteries helped the North Vietnamese counter American air strikes, as American supplies of mobile Stinger anti-aircraft missiles helped rebels in Afghanistan.

Let us now return to the concept of symmetrical and asymmetrical warfare. Recall that symmetrical wars involve opposing forces with significant similarities in key areas like force sizes, organizational systems, and levels of technology. In some cases of symmetry, the superiority of one side's resources and doctrine emerged to produce a quick victory. The two best examples are Great Britain's victory over Argentina in the Falkland Islands War (1982) and the American-led coalition victory over Iraq in the Persian Gulf War (1991). In both cases, markedly superior training, doctrine, economic resources, and technology led to quick victories with relatively light casualties for the victors.

The Arab-Israeli Wars (especially that of 1967) are another case in point. Arab and Israeli military systems were both modeled on those of the superpowers, who gave or sold sophisticated military technology to both sides; the Israelis were closely allied to the United States, the Arab states were normally allied to the Soviet Union. Superior Israeli motivation, training, and American-built weapons systems allowed Israel to defeat much larger Arab coalitions. In 1967, Israel humbled a coalition of Egypt, Jordan, and Syria in just six days. Egypt alone suffered 11,500 dead and lost 264 combat aircraft, many of them destroyed on the ground on the first day. By contrast Israel lost 800 dead and just forty combat aircraft. In all, Israel inflicted battlefield deaths at a rate of eighteen to one; destroyed tanks at a rate of ten to one; and achieved an air combat kill ratio of twenty-five to one.

In some cases, the opposing forces were symmetrical, but neither had a distinct advantage over the other. In these cases, wars were often protracted and failed to reach permanent settlements. Between 1950 and 1953, the Korean War was one such conflict. South Korea defended an attack by North Korea in 1950 with the help of United Nations forces led by the United States. When UN forces crossed into North Korea and continued to move north, China entered the war. Chinese numerical superiority met UN technological superiority as the front returned to a line nearly contiguous with the pre-1950 border. Throughout 1952 and 1953, the two sides fought a bloody and inconclusive war that yielded a cease-fire but to this day still lacks a final treaty. Tensions on the peninsula remain high, the United States still garrisons Korea, and, technically, the two Koreas remain at war.

The extremely brutal Iran-Iraq War (1980–1988) is another case in point. Iraq, which was supported by Kuwaiti and Saudi money, had modern Soviet and western weapons. Iran, in the midst of an Islamic revolution, had higher morale and a larger population base. Neither side was able to overwhelm the other, despite repeated attempts to do so. The eight-year war may have cost as many as 1,500,000 lives. The death toll included tens of thousands of civilians as both sides used long-range artillery and poison gas to attack civilian centers. As in Korea, a cease-fire stopped the killing, but no permanent treaty followed. Tensions between the two nations remain high.

These wars were also, in part, legacies of decolonization combined with Cold War tensions. Iran and Iraq, long dominated by the British and French, struggled to develop independently of the nations of western Europe. The Islamic revolution of 1978 in Iran was partly a protest against continued western intrusion into the internal affairs of that state. The kidnapping of fifty-two Americans in Iran for 444 days symbolized both an anti-western theme in the Iranian revolution and the fact that the United States, which had supported the unpopular Shah out of a desire to form anti-Soviet alliances in the region, had replaced Britain and France as the target of popular anger.

The complex interplay of decolonization and the Cold War also played a key role in one of the classical asymmetrical wars of the twentieth century, Vietnam. The Vietnam War is in fact two wars, the one France fought from 1947 to 1954 and the one the United States fought against the same opponent from 1965 to 1973. For France, recolonization of Vietnam was a key component to reconstructing its empire in the wake of their defeat in World War II. Great Britain, charged with accepting the Japanese surrender in the southern half of the country, quickly helped the French reestablish their authority, going so far as to use former Japanese prisoners of war on France's behalf. Britain fought for the principle of recolonization because it too was facing the challenge of reestablishing control in parts of its empire. In the northern half of Vietnam, Chinese forces quickly disarmed the Japanese then returned to China to fight in the civil war that had broken out there. As a result, Viet Minh guerrilla forces were able to establish a strong position in the north and declare Vietnam independent of France in 1947. From then until 1954, France fought an unsuccessful asymmetric war to defeat the Viet Minh, ending with the disaster at Dien Bien Phu.

The United States supported the French effort not out of sympathy for recolonization, but out of fear that the Viet Minh, and its charismatic leader, Ho Chi Minh, were tools of both Chinese and Soviet communism. Thus for the United States, Vietnam represented an important Cold War battleground. American advisers were later followed by the insertion of troops in 1965. At the height of the war, the United States had more than 500,000 men and millions of dollars of sophisticated equipment in Southeast Asia, but could not defeat the Vietnamese guerrillas. As Mao Tse-Tung had preached, the Vietnamese dragged the fighting out long enough for American popular opinion to turn against the war and in 1973 the United States completed a withdrawal of its troops.

The frustrations that the vastly wealthier and more complex United States military felt in Vietnam were repeated in other asymmetrical wars. France fought from 1954 to 1962 to keep its hold on Algeria, but the Algerian National Liberation Front (ALN) used strategies and tactics similar to those of guerrillas across the world to force the French out and turn popular opinion inside France against the war. By 1958, France itself seemed on the brink of civil war over the issue until Charles de Gaulle returned to the government and negotiated a peace settlement. As in Vietnam and many other asymmetrical wars, the French inflicted many more deaths than they suffered (10,000 French dead to 70,000 Algerian), but the determination of the ALN to continue the fight overcame French popular will.

For the wealthier power, winning asymmetrical wars required combining military force with programs of social and political reform that removed or ameliorated the worst aspects of colonialism. Many French and American leaders recognized this need, but had difficulty persuading local elites and their own governments to redistribute land or share power. In Malaysia in the 1950s, the British combined effective counter-insurgency operations with domestic reform to neutralize a communist uprising there. While the Americans recognized the role that such reforms played in defeating the communists, they failed to fully incorporate such plans in Vietnam.

Guerrilla wars also plagued Africa and Latin America in the post-war period. These conflicts were often fueled by American, European, and Soviet money. Thus Cold War motivations combined with local animosities and rivalries to create prolonged and bloody conflicts. The United States, concerned with what it alleged were communist insurgencies near its borders, devoted considerable energies and resources to conflicts in El Salvador, Nicaragua, and elsewhere. In Africa, similar patterns obtained. In Angola, Soviet and Cuban support of the Popular Movement for the Liberation of Angola produced a brutal civil war in the mid-1970s. The by-now familiar interplay of Cold War imperatives and local conditions fed local conflicts.

During the Cold War, the United States and the Soviet Union attempted to step into the power vacuums created by decolonization and the ebbing of European, especially British and French, power. In many cases, guerrilla groups proved successful in fending off the superpowers and attempts by Europeans to reassert their former colonial controls. The end of the Cold War has produced similar effects. In the former Soviet Union, Chechen rebels have strongly resisted Russian attempts to keep Chechnya under Russian rule. Guerrilla wars continue to plague poverty-stricken Africa as well, with terrible consequences for civilians caught in the crossfire.

The "collateral damage" that war inflicts on innocent people caught in the crossfire has led to several proposals, including a ban on land mines, which disproportionately injure and kill children. In another effort to limit the impact of war on civilians, western nations, especially the United States, have turned to aerial bombing and PGMs. Almost since its inception, proponents of aerial bombing have argued that precision air attacks can destroy military targets while leaving civilian targets unharmed, thus sparing innocent people from the dangers of warfare. Experiences since World War I have demonstrated to some that such neat parsing of military and civilian targets is simply impossible. Others put faith in technology's supposed ability to increase accuracy and precision targeting. The ultimate goal, avoiding civilian casualties, is noble, but maddeningly difficult to achieve.

Faith in precision appears to be a peculiarly American characteristic. One editorial cartoonist lampooned this obsession with a mock briefing given by a NATO spokesman after an attack during the air campaign over Yugoslavia in 1999. Spokesman: "NATO's attack on the convoy west of Pristina also resulted in the destruction of four APC's [armored personnel carriers] and a tank, which we do not regret and one red tractor, which we deeply regret. Also hit was a taxi, which we also regret, and a command car, which we don't. The highway was also damaged, much to our regret, except for the access road to the garrison, for which NATO does not apologize." Reporter: "Jamie, there are reports of shattered flower pots." Spokesman: "Would these be civilian flower pots?"[2]

Satire aside, it remains impossible for any weapons system to perfectly distinguish between military and civilian targets. Human error still exists, as it did when American warplanes accidentally struck the Chinese embassy in Belgrade. Tellingly, the Americans claimed that their technology was not to blame; instead they claimed that they targeted the wrong building because they were operating with faulty maps. In this case, the casualties were not just civilian, but official representatives of a non-belligerent nation. In other cases, legitimate military targets are located extremely close to civilian ones, either by happenstance or by design. The Americans accused Saddam Hussein of using his people as human shields during the Gulf War, placing civilians inside military facilities in the hope of deterring an air attack. Despite all of the best intentions, civilians continue to suffer during war and no solution on the horizon promises to eliminate that harsh reality.

Legacies

It is perhaps too soon to gauge accurately the legacy of the Cold War period. One clear legacy is the military role played by anti-imperial forces in Vietnam, Algeria, and elsewhere. They visibly demonstrated how much the military relationship between Europe and the rest of the world had changed. They also challenged the two recognized superpowers, the United States and the Soviet Union. They visibly demonstrated a point we have seen time and again: having presumed advantages in military organization and technology does not automatically equate into invincibility. In many parts of the world, guerrilla groups still pose a threat to larger, better financed militaries.

The legacy of nuclear weapons is equally unclear. Recently, the world's most powerful nations have attempted to stop the proliferation of atomic weapons technology across the globe. Whether they will be successful in the long run is still in doubt. Many states that lack such weapons would like to acquire them and are willing to defy international treaties and conventions to do so.

Finally, in the absence of the Cold War, many states have been forced to justify high defense expenditures. Some politicians have echoed British Prime Minister Tony Blair's statement that the post-Cold War world will be characterized by what Blair called an "imperialism of morality." In other words, the great powers will use their military strength to defend those who cannot defend themselves. Critics allege that the western powers use their force where it benefits them economically (Iraq) or where they want to punish a rogue European leader (Kosovo) but not where the suffering is indeed greatest (Rwanda).

All of these developments will doubtless affect the future of warfare and the future of the United States' presumptive role as the world's only remaining superpower. The superiority of American military technology will not automatically serve the nation well in the face of determined enemies, especially in asymmetrical wars. The end of the Cold War has not made the world a safer place. Indeed, people in Sub-Saharan Africa and the Middle East have seen few benefits to the end of the American–Soviet rivalry. Despite international efforts to curb warfare and its most deadly consequences, it would be foolish to presume that mankind will be any less warlike in the twenty-first century than it has been in earlier centuries. A careful study of the history of warfare is thus critical if this vital aspect of world history is to be understood.

Notes

1 Linda Grant De Pauw, *Battle Cries and Lullabies: Women in War From Prehistory to the Present* (Norman: University of Oklahoma Press, 1998), p. 293.
2 G. B. Trudeau, *Buck Wild Doonesbury* (Kansas City: Andrews McMeel, 1999), p. 151.

Further reading

On guerrilla warfare see Edward E. Rice, *Wars of the Third Kind: Conflict in Underdeveloped Countries* (Berkeley: University of California Press, 1988) and John Shy and Thomas W. Collier, "Revolutionary War," in Peter Paret, ed., *Makers of Modern Strategy from Machiavelli to the Nuclear Age* (Princeton: Princeton University Press, 1986). On women and warfare, see Linda Grant De Pauw, *Battle Cries and Lullabies: Women in War From Prehistory to the Present* (Norman: University of Oklahoma Press, 1998) and, for the American side, Jeanne Holm, *Women in the Military: An Unfinished Revolution* (Novato, CA: Presidio Press, revised edition, 1993). For Vietnam there are many good books. Among the best are Neil Sheehan, *A Bright Shining Lie: John Paul Vann and America in Vietnam* (New York: Random House, 1988) and George Herring, *America's Longest War: The United States and Vietnam, 1950–1975* (New York: Knopf, 1986). On the Cold War see Jeremy Isaacs and Taylor Downing, *Cold War: An Illustrated History, 1945–1991* (New York: Little, Brown, 1998), a companion to a Cable News Network series and Walter LaFeber, *America, Russia, and the Cold War, 1945–1992* (New York: McGraw-Hill, 1993), now in its seventh edition. For Africa fewer works exist, but see two new books, Christopher Clapham, ed., *African Guerillas* (Bloomington: Indiana University Press, 1998) and Anthony Clayton, *Frontiersmen: Warfare in Africa since 1950* (London: UCL Press, 1999).

Conclusions

Warfare is one of humankind's most difficult activities to fully understand. The very horror of warfare stands in stark contrast to what people want to believe about themselves and the societies they create. Many people thus try to place warfare in a separate category of abhorrent or abnormal behavior that is best understood as an exception or sideshow to humankind's otherwise peaceful progress.

But warfare cannot be separated from other activities in human history. Virtually all human societies have engaged in warfare in one form or another. For many of the world's most advanced societies, warfare has been a common, even central, theme. The developing world continues to be plagued by wars, civil and external, that have contributed to the ongoing problems of those societies. Much as we might hope that we can simply wish warfare away, it is unrealistic to suppose that mankind's violent history has stopped.

How then can we, as historians, explain and understand warfare? One common explanation is to look at warfare exclusively from the perspective of technology and resources. At their most simple, these explanations argue that societies with access to the "best" weapons, or larger quantities of weapons, win wars. As we have seen in the preceding chapters, technology does matter. The Aztecs had no answer to Spain's gunpowder weapons in the fifteenth and sixteenth centuries, nor did Japan have an answer to the atomic bombs that the United States dropped on Hiroshima and Nagasaki in 1945. Technology has surely played decisive roles at key points in military history.

Still, a "technological determinism" argument does not fully explain warfare. First, "better" technologies are not always immediately self-evident. As we have seen, gunpowder weapons, which appear so dominant in retrospect, took a long time to become fully integrated into armed forces. To take a contemporary example, the United States is today debating the relative merits of constructing and deploying a missile defense system capable of destroying incoming enemy warheads. To its proponents, this technology is clearly "better" in that it promises to protect the United States from enemy attack. To its critics, however, such a system is the wrong technology because it leaves other methods of warhead delivery, such as a terrorist attack, undefended.

At this point, there is no way of knowing if this technology will "work" as its designers intend.

Furthermore, "better" technologies do not always win wars. Few people would have disagreed that in 1965 the United States enjoyed a tremendous technological superiority over its Vietnamese enemies. Still, these technologies were ill-suited for the war the United States was fighting. Moreover, structural flaws inside the American system negated any presumed advantages in American technology. Superior technology does not always guarantee victory.

If technology alone is insufficient, so is an exclusive focus on elite leadership. For many years military history focused an inordinate degree of attention on generals, admirals, and civilian leaders. Generalship is, of course, important to military history, but it alone is not the whole story. Since the 1970s historians have begun to analyze in greater detail the motivations, performance, and belief systems of "common" soldiers. To understand the history of warfare, one must study both the commanders and those they commanded.

It would be foolish to suggest that individuals are irrelevant to the history of warfare. But in order to understand an individual's role, one must understand his or her environment and the context within which he or she operated. Napoleon, brilliant though he surely was, could never have accomplished what he did without the achievements of the French Revolution and, ironically, the military innovations of the *Ancien régime* system that he helped to topple. Similarly, a Chinese general of Napoleonic abilities may have existed in 1894, but the backwardness of the Chinese military system would have prevented him from reversing the humiliating defeat his country suffered at the hands of the Japanese.

Much of military history is written with the intent of explaining why the winners won and the losers lost. This approach makes perfect sense for students of the battlefield and for men and women charged with studying past battles in order to improve their chances in future battles. But such an approach serves us less well. In this volume we have been less interested in explaining victory and defeat than in explaining the role and nature of warfare in global history. We therefore need another way to contextualize and analyze war.

For warfare to make sense in the larger realms of history, we must connect it to larger world history themes. Of these, four stand out as most important: epidemiology and germ transmission; processes of diffusion and syncretism; the "rise of the west"; and the industrial revolution. All of these themes have impacted the history of warfare and all have, in turn, been affected by warfare.

Many Europeans believed that their rapid conquest of the Americas was due to superior intelligence and divine will. We know now that the Europeans were carrying an important, invisible ally with them. Diseases like smallpox and measles, to which the Europeans had built up immunities over the centuries, left Native American communities far weaker than they would otherwise have been. By some estimates, disease killed ninety-five per cent of some native communities. To be sure, the advantages of European military technology were important as well, but tiny microbes killed far more enemy warriors than did bullets.

By contrast, Europeans had epidemiological problems in Africa where diseases like malaria and yellow fever decimated Europeans. As a result, European technological advantages did not result in colonization of Africa as quickly as they did in the Americas. Europeans had to wait until medical science provided cures or vaccinations for African diseases before they could put their military advantages to full use. Contemporaries did not understand the historical experiences that had created such a disease environment, but it nevertheless impacted the history of the wars they fought. We must, therefore, link warfare to this larger, often misunderstood, theme in global history. European imperialism was surely a function of European military advantages, but the scale and scope of imperialism also owes much to differing patterns of immunity and disease.

Global processes of cultural diffusion and syncretism also connect nicely to warfare. Many important military technologies have transferred relatively easily across civilization boundaries. The most famous example is gunpowder, developed, ironically enough, around the ninth century by Chinese chemists trying to find a potion for immortality. Gunpowder found its way to the Islamic Middle East and then to Europe, where it found a climate distinctly receptive to its potential for military use.

As in economics, society, and culture, some civilizations proved to be more adept at selectively adapting military ideas. Between 1853 and 1894, Japan demonstrated a remarkable ability to borrow military ideas from western Europe. Japan modeled its navy on Great Britain's unparalleled Royal Navy and its army on that of Prussia. Japan used its tradition of selective borrowing to create the strongest military force in East Asia. China, on the other hand, with less developed traditions of syncretism, held to outdated, but distinctly Chinese, ideas of the proper role and organization of a military. When the two met on the battlefield, Japan easily vanquished China.

Similarly, during the reign of Peter the Great (1672–1725), Russia undertook a massive program of selective adaptation from western Europe. Peter introduced western culture, dress, technology, and educational styles to Russia. He also undertook military reforms on the western model, giving Russia a modern fleet and a capable army of more than 300,000 men. He also constructed armaments factories, opened military schools, and imported western military manuals for study by his generals and admirals. These reforms made Russia a significant power in European affairs.

Understanding the "rise of the west" is impossible without looking at western advances in military organization. Between 1400 and 1600, western Europe underwent a "military revolution" that rapidly changed the nature and capabilities of Europeans in relation to non-Europeans. Gunpowder weapons, centralized financial and political systems, and population expansion gave Europeans the military advantages that allowed them to enforce their imperial will across the globe. Of course, the rise of the west had roots in economic, political, social, and cultural changes, but to ignore the military dimension is a serious mistake. European desires to colonize and dominate large parts of the globe translated into imperialism because of the military ability of European nations.

Industrialization is the fourth and final theme in world history that we shall explore in this conclusion. The industrial revolution provided societies like Great Britain, Germany, France, Japan, the Soviet Union, and the United States with the means to mass-produce identical (and thus built of interchangeable parts) weapons and ancillary technologies like railroads, telegraphs, and automobiles. Those societies that lacked industry were often at significant disadvantages. Furthermore, military and industrial mindsets often merged. The railroad industry, for example, borrowed the military concept of staff (those who do the planning) and line (those who do the work). Since the nineteenth century, many officers have moved smoothly from military careers into civilian industry.

Thus I hope that this book demonstrates the importance of warfare to any serious study of world history. If one assumes, as I did earlier in this conclusion, that warfare will remain a feature of human society, then an understanding of the history of warfare is not merely academic. Rather, history is crucial to the search for ways to mitigate and limit the worst features of war. It should also serve as a horrible warning to those who lightly or casually endorse war.

French historian Marc Bloch was a veteran of both world wars. In 1940, well past the age at which he would have been required to fight, he left his job at the Sorbonne and, for the second time, volunteered for the French army to repel German invaders. After the fall of France, Bloch (who was Jewish) continued his struggle in the French Resistance. Before the Germans tortured and executed him in 1944, he wrote a "statement of evidence" explaining why he thought his country had fared so poorly in 1940. Bloch blamed, among many factors, a failure of the French people to fully understand its own history and that of Europe more generally.

Bloch argued that "By examining how and why yesterday differed from the day before, [history] can reach conclusions which will enable it to foresee how tomorrow will differ from yesterday. The traces left by past events never move in a straight line, but in a curve that can be extended into the future."[1] Your job, as students of history, is to study the curved lines left by thousands of years of warfare and use them to better understand the world you live in today. If you succeed in doing so, you will have accomplished a difficult, but worthy, goal.

Note

1 Marc Bloch, *Strange Defeat: A Statement of Evidence Written in 1940* (New York: W. W. Norton, 1999), p. 118.

Index

Abbasid Caliphate, 29
Adrianople, Battle of, 19
Afghanistan, 87, 88, 93
Africa, 52, 101
  in Cold War era to present, 88, 89,
    93–97
  in nationalist and industrialist era,
    56–57
  in World War I, 62–72
Agincourt, Battle of, 28, 31
air warfare
  in Cold War era to present, 90–92,
    96
  in World War I, 62–65, 68, 70–71
  in World War II, 74–78, 80
aircraft carriers, 79
airplanes (*See* air warfare)
Akbar the Great, 42
Alexander the Great, 8, 11, 14, 16, 17
Algeria, 95
Alsace-Lorraine, 61, 66–67
American Civil War, 50, 52–55, 57
American Revolution, 40, 44, 47–48,
    51
Amerindians, 42, 44, 100–101
Amiens, Battle of, WWI, 70
amphibious operations, 82
Anatolia, 21, 22
Angola, 88, 95–96
Antioch, 31
Anzacs, 59, 62
Anzio, Battle of, WWII, 82
Aqaba, Battle of, WWI, 69
Aquinas, Thomas, 24
Arabia (*See also* Saudi Arabia), 68–69
Arab–Israeli Wars, 91, 93

archeological/anthropological evidence
    of early warfare, 7
archery (*See* arrow design; bows;
    crossbows)
Argentina, 93
Armenia, 21
armies (*See* military organization for
    warfare)
armor, 14, 15, 16, 17, 26, 40
armored personnel carriers (APC), 96
arrow design, 26–27
Arslan, Alp, 21
Art of War, The, 12
Arthasatra, 13, 20
artillery, 39–40
  in gunpowder weapon era, 41–43
  in nationalist and industrialist era,
    51–52
  in World War I, 63, 69
Asia, 3, 93
asymmetrical wars, 86, 93–95
Athens, 15, 17–18
Atlantic Wall, of WWII, 1
atomic bomb and nuclear weapons, 5,
    76, 80, 83–84, 90–91, 97, 99
Austerlitz, Battle of, 54
Australia, 59–72, 79
Austria, 50, 54, 59–72
Austro–Prussian War, 63
automatic weapons, 52
axes, 14, 16
Ayn Jalut, Battle of, 30
Aztecs, 7–8, 41–42, 99

Babur, 42
Balkans, World War I, 61

ballistas, 16
Barbarossa, Frederick (Holy Roman Emperor), 30
Barbarossa Jurisdiction Decree, 75
Bartov, Omer, 75
Battle of Britain, 79
battleships (See also naval warfare), 65–66
Bavaria, 49
Béatrice, Battle of, 85
Belarus, 92
Belgium, 59–72
Belgrade, 96
Berlin, 83
Bhagavad Gita, 18
Big Bertha, 63
biological weapons, 27, 93
Blair, Tony, 97
Blitzkreig, 80–81
Bloch, Marc, 102
blockades, 55
Boer War, 50, 57, 86
Bolshevism, 70, 71
bombards, 39
bombers, 5, 65, 74, 76, 77, 80, 90
bows, 14, 16, 21, 22, 23, 25, 26, 32
Braddock, Edward, 44
Brazil, 93
breech loading rifles, 51
Breitenfeld, Battle of, 42
British Expeditionary Force, 56
bronze weapons, 19
Browning machine guns, 64
Brusilov, Alexei, 61–62
bushido, 3, 19, 29
Byzantine Empire, 21–23, 32

cadets, 38
Cambrai, Battle of, WWI, 66
Canada, 60–72
Cannae, Battle of, 18
cannon (See artillery)
capitalism, 78
Caporetto, Battle of, WWI, 69, 70
Carthage, 15
castles (See also fortifications and defensive works), 27–28, 31
catapults, 16

cavalry
    in classical age, 11, 12, 13, 16–19
    in post-classical period, 21–23, 26, 28–33
Celts, 3
Central/Latin America, 88, 93, 95
Central Powers, World War I, 59
centralized government and military, 38, 45
Chaeroneia, Battle of, 17–18
Chail Nashim, 89
chariots, 13, 16, 18–19
Charles V of France, 31
Charles V of Spain, 36, 42
Chechnya, 96
chemical weapons, 93
chevauchées, 31
Ch'i Chi-kuang, 37
China, 3, 8, 100, 101
    in classical age, 12–17, 19, 20
    in Cold War era to present, 87, 88, 94, 95
    in gunpowder weapon era, 37, 39–41
    in nationalist and industrialist era, 46, 56
    nuclear capability of, 90
    in post-classical period, 25, 29, 30, 32
    in World War II, 75, 79
China Sea, Battle of, WWII, 81
Ch'ing Dynasty, 40
chivalry, 3, 19, 22, 29
Churchill, John (Duke of Marlborough), 38, 43
Churchill, Winston, 59–60
Citadelle du Québec, 34–35, 40
citizen-soldiers, 4, 10–12, 48
city-states of ancient Greece, 17
civilian casualties, 74–76, 91, 96
classical age (to 500 CE), 3, 9–20
    Alexander the Great in, 11, 14, 16–17
    battles of, 17–19
    cavalry in, 11, 12, 13, 16–19
    in China, 12–17, 19, 20
    discipline during, 12, 13, 19–20
    fortification and defensive works of, 11, 13, 15–16

in Greece, 9–12, 15, 17
Hannibal and, 18
in India, 13, 16–20
infantry in, 10–14, 16, 19
legacies of, 19–20
legions of Rome in, 15
military organization in, 10–11, 19–20
naval warfare in, 15, 20
in Persian Empire, 9–10, 14, 17
religion and warfare in, 19
in Rome, 11–12, 15, 17, 19, 20
rules of engagement in, 19
soldiers and commanders of, 10–14
Thermopylae in, 9, 13, 17, 18
weapons of, 14–17, 19
Clemanceau, Georges, 71
Colbert, Jean Baptiste, 38
Cold Harbor, Battle of, 55
Cold War era to present, 3, 85–98
air warfare in, 90–92, 96
Arab–Israeli Wars in, 91, 93
atomic bomb and nuclear weapons in, 90–91, 97
battles of significance in, 93–97
communications technology in, 92
computer technology in, 91–92
conscription/draft and, 89
Cuban Missile Crisis in, 91
Dien Bien Phu (1953–54) in, 85–86, 95
end of, 89
Falkland Island Wars in, 93
guerrilla warfare in, 85–91, 93, 95–96
Indochina and Vietnam in, 85–86
Iran Hostage Crisis in, 94
Iran–Iraq War in, 94
Korean War in, 94
legacies of, 97
medical advances, 92
military organization in, 86, 91–95, 97
missile weapons in, 90–92
morals and ethics of war in, 97
North Atlantic Treaty Organization (NATO) and, 89, 93, 96
Persian Gulf War in, 93, 96–97

smart weapons development, 91
soldiers and commanders in, 86–90
superpowers of, 92
"total war" and, 88
United Nations and, 94
Warsaw Pact and, 89, 93
weapons and machines of, 90–93
women in military during, 89–90
collateral damage (See civilian casualties)
colonialism, 74, 87, 100–101
commanders (See soldiers and commanders)
communications technology, 15–16, 53, 77, 92
Communism, 78, 95
composite bows, 26
computer technology, 91–92
condottieri, 32
Confederacy (See American Civil War)
Congo, 88
conscription/draft, 4, 5, 48
in Cold War era to present, 89
in World War I, 60
in World War II, 77
Constantinople, 28, 38, 39, 40, 41, 59
contingency planning, 50
Coral Sea, Battle of, 79
Crécy, Battle of, 28, 31
Crimean War, 51, 53
Cromwell, Oliver, 38
crossbows, 14–15, 26–28
cruise missiles, 91
Crusades, 3, 22, 23, 24, 27, 30–33
Cuba, 95
Cuban Missile Crisis, 91
cultural issues, 3, 35, 101

Damascus, Battle of, WWI, 69
D-Day, 1–2, 6, 81–83
Declaration of Paris, 55
defensive works (See fortification and defensive works)
Demetrius of Rhodes, 16
Denmark, 50
Dien Bien Phu (1953–54), 85–86, 95
discipline in armed forces
in classical age, 12, 13, 19–20

in gunpowder weapon era, 36–37, 41, 44

in nationalist and industrialist era, 46

in post-classical period, 23

disease as aid/hindrance to colonial expansion, 100–101

doctrinal development, 50

draft (*See* conscription/draft)

Dreadnoughts, 65–66

drill tactics, 36–37

Ducas, John, 21–22

Easchylus, 10

economic issues of war, 3, 101–102

in gunpowder weapon era, 35, 38, 40–41

in World War I, 70

in World War II, 78–79

Edward III of England, 31

Egypt, modern-day, 93, 93–94

Einsatzgruppen, 75

Einstein, Albert, 80

Eisenhower, Dwight D., 1–2, 5

El Salvador, 95

Elizabeth I of England, 42

Ellis, John, 64

engineering (*See* fortifications and defensive works)

England and Great Britain, 54, 86, 101, 102

in Cold War era to present, 87, 93, 94, 95, 96, 97

in gunpowder weapon era, 34–35, 38, 40, 41, 42

in nationalist and industrialist era, 47–50, 52, 53, 56–57

nuclear capability of, 90

in post-classical period, 31

in World War I, 59–72

in World War II, 74–84

English Civil War, 43

Enigma machine, 79

Enlightenment, 6, 43, 48

Eritrea, 88

Ethiopia, 88

Faisal, Emir, 69

Falkenhayn, Erich von, 69

Falkland Island Wars, 93

Fascism, 71, 78

Fermi, Enrico, 80

feudalism, 22–25, 31

flame throwers, 66, 70–71

Flanders, Battle of, WWI, 68

flintlocks, 40, 43

Foch, Ferdinand, 62, 70, 71

fortifications and defensive works, 15–16, 27–28

in classical age, 11, 13, 15–16

in gunpowder weapon era, 37, 39, 40–41, 43

in nationalist and industrialist era, 55

France, 40, 102

in Cold War era to present, 94–96

in gunpowder weapon era, 34–35, 38, 42, 43

Indochina and Vietnam and, 85–87, 94–95

in nationalist and industrialist era, 48, 50, 52

nuclear capability of, 90

in post-classical period, 31

in World War I, 59–72

in World War II, 77–84

Franco–Prussian War, 69

Franklin, Benjamin, 40

Frederick the Great of Prussia, 43–44

Fredericksburg, Battle of, 55

French and Indian Wars, 44

French Foreign Legion, 89

French Resistance, WWII, 2, 102

French Revolution, 48, 53, 100

Galliéni, Joseph Simon, 67

Gallipoli (1915), 59–60, 62, 82

Gatling guns, 52

de Gaulle, Charles, 95

general staff system, 50

Geneva Accords, 86

Geneva Convention, 3, 55

Genghis Khan, 6, 23

German Unification, Wars of, 53

Germany, 102

in gunpowder weapon era, 43

in nationalist and industrialist era, 50
in World War I, 59–72
in World War II, 73–84
Gettysburg, Battle of, 51, 55
Giap, Vo Nguyen, 85–86
gladius, 15, 18
Gotha bombers, 65, 77
Grant De Pauw, Linda, 90
Great Britain (*See* England and Great Britain)
Great Wall of China, 8, 12, 13, 16
Greece (*See also* classical age), 3, 9–12, 15, 17, 41, 62
Guderian, Heinze, 66
Guernica, 75–76
guerrilla warfare, 85–91, 93, 95–96
gunpowder weapon era, 3, 34–45, 51, 99, 101–102
American Revolution and, 40, 44
artillery and, 40–43
Asian nations in, 35
battles of significance in, 41–44
centralized government and military in, 38, 45
in China, 37, 39, 40, 41
cultural issues of, 35
danger of early designs in, 39
development of, 39, 40, 44
discipline of military and, 36–37, 41, 44
drill tactics in, 36–37
economic issues and, 35, 38, 40–41
in England, 34–35, 38, 40–43
Enlightenment in, 43
fortifications and defensive works of, 39–41, 43
inaccuracy of aim in early weapons, 40
in France, 34–35, 38, 40, 42, 43
in India, 34, 42, 44
infantry and, 40
in Islamic nations, 36, 37, 38, 39, 41
in Japan, 36, 37, 41
legacies of, 44–45
military organization in, 36–38, 42–45
militia in, 35, 38

Napoleon and, 38
naval warfare in, 41
in Ottoman Empire, 39, 40, 41, 42
political issues in, 35, 38
and post-classical period, 28, 30
professional soldiers and standing armies of, 36, 42
in Prussia, 43–44
Québec (1759) and, 34–35, 37, 44
religion and warfare in, 42, 43
resistance to gunpowder weapons and, 36, 37
rules of engagement in, 43
siege warfare in, 35, 39
social issues in, 35, 37
soldiers and commanders in, 35–38
Thirty Years War in, 37, 39, 42–43
veteran's support in, 38
weapons of, 39–41
Gupta Empire (*See* India)
Gupta, Chandra, 13, 16
Gupta, Samudra, 13
Gustavus Adolphus of Sweden, 37, 42

Hadrian's wall, 16
Hague Conference, 3, 55
Haig, Douglas, 32, 67–68
Han Dynasty, 12, 13, 17, 20, 29
Hannibal, 18
Hanson, Victor Davis, 17
Heihachiro, Togo, 46–47
helepolis, 16
helicopters, 92
Henry VIII of England, 41
Hiroshima, 76, 99
history of war, 6–8, 99
HMS Victory, 41
Ho Chi Minh, 83, 95
Hobbes, Thomas, 6, 7
Hoffman, Max, 67
Holland, 42, 81
Holocaust, 75
Holy Land, 22
Holy Roman Empire, 42
Hong Kong, 56
hoplites, 14, 17
hoplons, 14
horseshoes, 22

hostages and ransom, 23
Hôtel des Invalides, 38
Hundred Years War, 31
Hungary, 59–72
Hussein, Sadam, 96–97

Ibn-Munqidh, Usamah, 27
imperialism, 74, 100–101
India
    in classical age, 13, 16, 17–20
    in Cold War era to present, 87, 93
    in gunpowder weapon era, 34, 40,
        42, 44
    in nationalist and industrialist era,
        53
    nuclear capability of, 90
    in post-classical period, 24–26, 29,
        30, 32–33
    in World War I, 60–72
    in World War II, 83
Indochina and Vietnam, 83, 85–87, 89,
    91, 93–95, 100
industrialization (See also nationalist and
    industrialist era), 3, 46–58, 102
infantry
    in classical age, 10, 11, 13–14, 16,
        19
    in gunpowder weapon era, 40
    in post-classical period, 21–22, 24,
        28–33
intelligence gathering, 13, 50, 79–80
Intercontinental Ballistic Missiles
    (ICBMs), 90
internet, 92
Intifada, 87
Iran Hostage Crisis, 94
Iran–Iraq War, 94
Iraq, 93, 97
Irish Republican Army, 87
iron weapons, 19
Isandhlwana, Battle of, 56–57
Islamic (Muslim) nations (See also
    Crusades)
    in gunpowder weapon era, 36, 37–41
    in post-classical period, 21–23, 30,
        32
Israel, 89, 90, 93–94
Italy, 27, 32, 39, 61–72, 77–84

Jackson, Thomas "Stonewall," 55
James II of Scotland, 39
janissaries (See also Islamic nations), 38,
    41
Japan, 3, 99, 100, 101, 102
    in Cold War era to present, 94
    in gunpowder weapon era, 36, 37, 41
    in nationalist and industrialist era,
        46–47, 52, 56
    in post-classical period, 24, 26–29
    in World War II, 75–84, 87
javelins, 14, 16, 18
Jericho, 31
Jerusalem, 31
Jihads, 3
Joan of Arc, 31
Joffre, Joseph, 61, 67
de Jomini, Antoine Henri, 54–55
Jordan, 93–94
Jourdan Law, 48
Julius Caesar, 8, 12, 86
"just war" theory, 24
Jutland, Battle of, WWI, 66

Kafartab Castle, Crusades, 27
Kazakhstan, 92
Kemal, Mustafa, 59–60, 62
King George's (of England) War, 43, 44
von Kluck, Alexander, 67
knights, 22–23, 26, 30, 36, 37
ko, 14, 16
Kondor Legion, 75–76
Korea, 29, 75, 93, 94
Korean War, 94
Kosovo, 97
Kuwait, 94

Lancaster bomber, 76
lances, 22
landing craft, 5, 82
Lateran Council, 26–27
Latin America (See Central/Latin
    America)
Lawrence, T.E., 68–69, 86–87
legality of war, 2–3
legions of Rome, 15
legitimacy of war, 2–3
Lend-Lease Program, WWII, 78–79

Lenin, Illya, 73
Leonidas, 9–10
Lepanto, Battle of, 41
Lettow-Vorbeck, Paul von, 68
Leuthen, Battle of, 43–44
Levée en Masse, 48
li, 3, 19, 29
Liberty aircraft engine, 77
Liverpool Pals, World War I, 62
longboats, 29
longbows, 28, 31, 32, 40
Louis XIV of France, 38
Ludendorff Offensives, 69, 70
Lusitania, 65, 74

Macedonia, 11, 14, 17–18
machine guns, 52, 64, 66
MAGIC, 78–79
Maginot Line, 81
Magna Carta, 23
Mainz, Siege of, 43
malaria, 101
Malaysia, 95
Malplaquet, Battle of, 43
mamluks (*See also* Islamic nations), 36,
    37, 41
Manchu (Ch'ing Dynasty), 31, 40
Manhattan Project (*See also* atomic
    bomb), 80
Manila, Battle of, WWII, 82, 83
Manstein, Erich von, 75
Manzikert (1071), 21–22, 30
Mao Tse-Tung, 12, 88
Maori, 7
Marathon, Battle of, 9, 10
"March to the Sea," Sherman's, 55
Marengo, Battle of, 54
Market Garden project, 81
Marne, Battle of, WWI, 67, 70
Marshall, George, 20
Martel, Charles, 25, 30
mass production of weapons, 50–51
Masurian Lakes, Battle of, WWI, 67
matchlock rifles, 39–40
Maurice of Nassau, 36–37
Maxim, Hiram, 52
measles, 100
medical advances, 15, 62, 70, 92

Medieval Europe (*See* post-classical era)
Mehmet II, 38
mercenaries, 4, 21, 32, 36, 42–43
Meso-America, 3
Mexico, 79
midair refueling, 92
Middle East, Cold War era to present,
    93, 97
Midway, Battle of, WWII, 78–79
military organization, 4, 6–8, 100–102
    asymmetrical wars and, 86, 93–95
    in classical age, 10–11, 19–20
    in Cold War era to present, 86,
        91–95, 97
    in gunpowder weapon era, 36–38,
        42–45
    in nationalist and industrialist era,
        47–50
    in post-classical period, 23, 28, 32
    symmetrical wars and, 86, 93–95
    in World War II, 77
militias, 4, 35, 38, 48
Millis, Walter, 47
mines, 27
minié balls, 51
missile weapons, 14, 16, 17, 21, 39,
    90–92, 99
Mogadishu, 88
Moguls, 40, 42
Mongols, 22, 23, 25, 29–32
Mons Meg, 39
Montcalm, Marquis de, 34–35, 37
Montgomery, Bernard, 77
Montigny Mitrailleuse, 52
Moors, 30
moral and ethical issues, 2–3, 13, 24,
    60, 97
musketeers, 37, 43
muskets, 37, 43, 51
Muslims (*See* Islamic nations)
Mutually Assured Destruction (MAD),
    90
muzzle loading rifles, 51

Nagasaki, 76, 80, 99
Nanking, 75
Napoleon, 5, 38, 48–55, 57, 86, 100
nationalist and industrialist era, 46–58

in Africa, 56–57
American Civil War and, 50, 52, 53, 55, 57
American Revolution and, 47–48
aristocracy vs. democracy in, 49
artillery in, 51–52
battles of significance of, 53–57
Boer War in, 50, 57
in China, 46, 56
communications technology in, 53
discipline of armies in, 46
in England, 47–57
Enlightenment and, 48
fortifications and defensive works of, 55
in France, 48, 50, 52
French Revolution and, 48, 53
general staff system and, 50
ideological and societal reforms of, 47, 49
in India, 53
in Japan, 46–47, 52, 56
legacies of, 57–58
mass production of weapons in, 50–51
military organization in, 47–50
militias in, 48
Napoleon and, 48–57
naval warfare in, 46–47, 52, 56
pacifism vs. warfare in, 55–56
professional soldiers and standing armies in, 49–50
in Prussia, 49–50, 52–56
railroad development and, 53
rifle development and, 51, 57
rules of engagement in, 55–58
in Russia, 46–47, 49, 50, 54
Russo–Japanese War in, 46, 50, 52, 56–57, 67
soldiers and commanders of, 47–50
Tsushima Straits (1905) in, 46–47, 56
weapons of, 50–53
Native Americans (See Amerindians)
naval warfare, 65–66, 101
    in classical age, 15, 20
    in gunpowder weapon era, 41

in nationalist and industrialist era, 46–47, 52, 56
in post-classical period, 29
in World War I, 59
in World War II, 79, 81
Nazism, 74–75
Neolithic civilization, 7
New Zealand, 59–72
Nicaragua, 95
Normandy Invasion and D-Day, 1–2, 6, 81–83
Normans, 27
North Atlantic Treaty Organization (NATO), 89, 93, 96
North Korea, 93
Norway, 81
nuclear weapons (See atomic bombs and nuclear weapons)

Okinawa, Battle of, WWII, 83
operations in war, definition of, 6
Opium Wars, 56
origins of war, 6–8
Ottoman Empire, 39, 40–42, 59–72
Overlord (See Normandy Invasion; D-Day)

P-51 fighters, 77
Pacific Theater of WWII, 82
pacifism vs. warfare, 13, 55–56
Pakistan, nuclear capability of, 90
Palestine (See also Crusades), 27, 30
    in Cold War era to present, 87
    in World War I, 68–69
Pals Battalions, World War I, 62
Panzer Corps, 66, 81
paratroopers, 81–82
Paris, 66–67, 69, 70
Paris Gun, 63
Passchendaele, Battle of, WWI, 68
patriotism, 60
Patton, George, 1, 77
Pearl Harbor, 79, 81, 82
Peloponnesian Wars, 20
Persian Empire, 9–10, 14, 17
Persian Gulf War, 93, 96–97
Peru, 89
Peter the Great of Russia, 101

Petersburg (US), Battle of, 55
phalanx formation, 11, 14, 17, 18
Philip Augustus of France, 27, 30
Philip II of Macedon, 17
Pickett's Charge (Gettysburg), 51, 55
pila, 15
Plan XVII (France), 61, 66–67
plunder, 23
poison gas, 15, 30, 63–64
Poitiers, Battle of, 28, 31
Poland, 75–84
political issues, 3, 8, 101–102
    in gunpowder weapon era, 35, 38
    in post-classical period, 29
    in World War I, 70
Popular Movement for the Liberation of
    Angola, 95–96
Port Arthur, Siege of, 46–47
Portugal, 42, 88
post-classical period (500–1450), 21–33
    battles of significance in, 28–32
    Byzantine Empire in, 21–23, 32
    cavalry in, 21–23, 26, 28–33
    China in, 25, 29, 30, 32
    chivalry in, 22
    Crusades in, 22–24, 27, 30–33
    discipline in, 23
    feudalism in, 22–25, 31
    fortifications and defensive structures
        in, 27–28
    gunpowder weapons in, 28, 30
    Hundred Years War in, 31
    India in, 29, 24–36, 30, 32–33
    infantry in, 21–22, 24, 28–33
    Islamic (Muslim) nations in, 21–23,
        30, 32
    Japan in, 24, 26–29
    legacies of, 32–33
    Manzikert (1071) in, 21–22, 30
    military organization in, 23, 28, 32
    Mongols and, 22–23, 25, 29, 30–32
    morals and ethics in, 24
    naval warfare in, 29
    political issues of, 29
    religion and warfare in, 21–22, 24,
        29, 30, 32
    Roman Empire in, 21–22, 29
    siege warfare in, 27, 29, 31

    soldiers and commanders of, 22–25
    Vikings and, 29
    weapons and machines of, 21–22,
        25–28
Precision Guided Munitions (PGMs),
    91, 92, 96
prisoners of war, 23
professional soldiers and standing
    armies, 4, 32, 36, 42, 49–50
Prussia, 43–44, 49–56, 101
Punic Wars, 15
Pydna, Battle of, 18

Qin Dynasty, 12, 16, 17
Québec (1759), 34–35, 37, 44

Racism, 74
radar, 5, 80
railroads, 53, 102
rapid-fire weapons, 52
Rassenkampf, 74
reasons for war, 7, 99
recruitment options (See also
    conscription), 4
Red Cross, 56
Reichenau, Walther von, 75
religion and warfare, 3, 7, 29
    in classical age, 19
    in gunpowder weapon era, 42, 43
    in post-classical period, 21–22, 24,
        30, 32
    in World War I, 60
Rennenkampf, Pavel, 67
repeating rifles, 57
resources and wars, 7
Rhodesia, 89
Richard I (Lionheart) of England, 27, 30
rifles, 39–40, 51, 57
Riga, Battle of, WWI, 69
"rise of the west," 101–102
road building, Roman, 15
Romanus, Emperor, 21–22
Rome, 3, 11–12, 15, 17, 19, 20–22, 29
Rommel, Erwin, 1, 77
Roosevelt, Franklin D., 78
Rousseau, Jean-Jacques, 6–7
rules of engagement, 3, 7
    in classical age, 19

in gunpowder weapon era, 43
in nationalist and industrialist era,
   55–58
Russia and Soviet Union, 29, 101, 102
   Afghanistan War and, 87, 88, 93
   in Cold War era to present, 87, 89,
      93, 96, 97
   collapse of Soviet Union and, 92
   in nationalist and industrialist era,
      46–47, 49, 50, 54
   nuclear capability of, 90
   Russo–Japanese War and, 46, 50,
      52, 56–57, 67
   in World War I, 59–72
   in World War II, 73–84
Russian Civil War, 70
Russian Revolution of 1905, 46
Russo–Japanese War, 46, 50, 52,
   56–57, 67
Rwanda, 88, 97

Sacred Band of Thebes, 17–18
St. Mihiel, Battle of, WWI, 65
Salamis, Battle of, 10
Samsonov, Aleksander, 67
samurai, 25, 26, 36, 37, 41
sapping, 27
sarissa, 14
Saudi Arabia, 94
Schlieffen Plan, 60–61, 66, 67
Schrecklichkeit (frightfulness), 66
Schutztruppe, 68
Second Coalition, War of, 54
secret service, 13
Seljuk Turks (*See also* Islamic nations),
   21, 32
sepoys (*See also* India), 44
Serbia, 61, 92
serpentine, 40
Seven Weeks War, 50
Seven Years War, 44, 48
shell shock, 62
Sherman, William, 55
shields, 14, 15, 16
Shining Path (*Sendero Luminoso*) rebels,
   89
Showalter, Dennis, 50, 58
siege warfare, 16, 27, 29, 31, 35, 39

Sino–Japanese Wars, 46, 50, 56
slings, 14
small arms, 39–40
smallpox, 100
smart weapons development, 91
smokeless powder, 51
Social Darwinism, 74
societal issues, 2–3
   in gunpowder weapon era, 35, 37
   in nationalist and industrialist era,
      47, 49
   in World War II, 74–75
soldiers and commanders, 100
   of classical age, 10–14
   of Cold War era to present, 86–90
   of gunpowder weapon era, 35–38
   of nationalist and industrialist era,
      47–50
   of post-classical period, 22–25
   of World War I, 60–63
   of World War II, 74–77
Somme, Battle of, WWI, 66
Song Dynasty, 25, 30, 32
South Africa, 90, 93
South Asia, 3
Soviet Union (*See* Russia and Soviet
   Union)
Spain, 39–41, 86, 99
Spanish–American War, 50
Spanish Armada, 41
Spanish Civil War, 75–76
Sparta, 9–11
spears, 14, 15, 16, 18, 25
Spring and Autumn Period, China, 12,
   13, 19
Stalin, Joseph, 1–2, 73
Stalingrad, 73–74
steam engines, 53
stirrups, 13, 22, 25–26, 30, 32
"storm troopers," 69
strategy in war, definition of, 6
submarines and U-boats, 65–66, 70–71,
   92
Sudan, 52
Sun Tzu, 12, 20, 88
superpowers, 83, 87, 92
Sweden, 37, 42
swords, 14, 15, 16, 18, 25, 26, 32

symmetrical wars, 86, 93–95
syncretism, 44, 101
Syria, 93–94

tactics in war, definition of, 6
Taiping Rebellion, 56
tank warfare, 66, 68, 70–71, 81–82
Tannenberg, Battle of, WWI, 67
Taranto, Battle of, WWII, 81
technological advances in warfare (See
    also weapons and machines of
    war), 2, 5–6
"technological determinism", 99–100
telegraphy, 53, 102
terrorism, 99
Tet Offensive, 88
Thebes, 17–18
Thermopylae, 9, 13, 17, 18
Thirty Years War, 37, 39, 42–43
Thucydides, 20
Tilly, John Tserclaes von, 42
Toltecs, 8
"total war," 66, 71, 88
trebuchet, 27
trench warfare, 61–63, 66, 68
triremes, 15
Truman, Harry, 84
Tsushima Straits (1905), 46–47, 56
Turkey, 21, 41, 59–72, 91
Tyre, 11

U-boats, 65–66, 70–71
Uganda, 88
Ukraine, 92
ULTRA, 79
United Nations, 94
United States, 49, 50, 102
    in Cold War era to present, 89,
        93–97
    nuclear capability of, 90
    Vietnam and, 86, 88, 91–95, 100
    in World War I, 63–72
    in World War II, 78–84
Urban II, Pope, 22

Valmy, Battle of, 53
de Vauban, Sébastien Le Prestre, 40–41,
    43

Venice, 41
Verdun, Battle of, WWI, 65, 69–70
Versailles Peace Conference, 69, 71
veteran's support, 38
Victoria Cross, 57
Viet Cong/Viet Mihn, 89, 95
Vietnam and Indochina, 83–95, 100
Vikings, 29
violence of warfare, 2–3
Visigoths, 19

War of the Austrian Succession, 44
Warring States Period, China, 19
Warsaw Pact, 89, 93
warships, 41
Washington, George, 44
weapons and machines of war, 5
    in classical age, 14–16, 17, 19
    in Cold War era to present, 90–93
    in gunpowder weapon era, 39–41
    in nationalist and industrialist era,
        50–53
    in post-classical period, 21–22,
        25–28
    "technological determinism" and,
        99–100
    in World War I, 63–66
    in World War II, 77–80
Wilson, Woodrow, 71
Wolfe, James, 34–35, 37, 51
Women Accepted for Volunteer
    Emergency Service (WAVES), 76
women in military, 4, 76–77, 89–90
Women's Airforce Service Pilots
    (WASP), 76
Women's Royal Navy Service (WRNS),
    76
World War I, 3, 6, 32, 41, 52, 56,
        59–72, 87
    air warfare in, 62–65, 68, 70–71
    artillery in, 63, 69
    battles of significance in, 66–70
    command structures in, 70
    economic issues of, 70
    fronts in, 68–60
    Gallipoli (1915) in, 59–60, 62
    legacies of, 70–71
    Ludendorff Offensives in, 69, 70

medical advances of, 62, 70
morals and ethics in, 60
naval warfare in, 59, 65–66, 70–71
Plan XVII (France) in, 61, 66–67
political issues of, 70
religion and warfare in, 60
Schlieffen Plan in, 60–61, 66, 67
soldiers and commanders in, 60–63
"storm troop" tactics in, 69
tank warfare in, 66, 68, 70–71
"total war" in, 66, 71
trench warfare in, 61–63, 66, 68
Versailles Peace Conference of, 69,
    71
weapons and machines of, 63–66
World War II, 3, 4, 5, 7, 20, 35, 73–84
air warfare in, 74–78, 80
atomic bomb and, 76, 80, 83–84
battles of significance in, 80–83
civilian casualties in, 74–76
communications technology in, 77
conscription/draft in, 77
decline of European military might
    in, 83
economic issues of, 78–79
Holocaust and, 75
ideological and societal issues of,
    74–75
intelligence gathering in, 79–80

Japan in, 87
legacies of, 83–84
Lend-Lease Program and, 78–79
"military globalism" in, 83
military organization of, 77
naval warfare in, 79, 81
Nazism and, 74–75
Normandy Invasion and D-Day in,
    1–2, 6, 81–83
Pacific Theater of, 82
paratroopers in, 81–82
radar in, 80
soldiers and commanders in, 74–77
Stalingrad in, 73–74
superpowers emergence in, 83
weapons and machines of, 77–80
women in military and, 76–77

Xenophon, 17, 20
Xerxes, 9

yellow fever, 101
Ypres, Battle of, WWI, 63, 64,
    67–68
Yugoslavia, 77, 96

Zhukov, Georgi, 73
Zimbabwe, 89
Zulus, 56–57